The Covid-19 Crisis in South

This edited book provides a range of perspectives on the handling of particular aspects of the Covid-19 pandemic across the principal states of South Asia.

As the first academic volume to deal with the Covid-19 pandemic in South Asia, it examines such issues as how India has dealt with the fallout of the pandemic on its substantial diaspora in the Middle East; the competitive Sino-Indian vaccine diplomacy strategies in Bangladesh; Nepal's attempts to cope with the pandemic, in light of its limited health infrastructure; Sri Lanka's differential treatment of its population based upon ethnic preferences; and how Pakistan's civil–military relations shaped its handling of the pandemic. The Introduction and the first section summarize the responses to the pandemic made by each principal state in the region. These chapters assess the process of decision-making within each state, with special attention placed on identifying and analzying the actors involved.

The Covid-19 pandemic is also reshaping international relations of the subcontinent, and the pandemic has laid bare several new cross-border challenges and opportunities that states will have to contend with in the future. The book also considers five of the most pressing issue areas. First, it considers how diaspora communities in the Gulf were affected by the pandemic, and what lessons South Asian sending states can take from protecting their citizens in the future. Second, the Covid-19 pandemic will affect how countries engage in status politics, shaping which countries will be able to lead in regional relations. Third, the Covid-19 pandemic is likely to affect prospects for regional cooperation, both for dealing with the current pandemic as well as future crises. Fourth, it will shape how South Asian states engage in global governance. Fifth, South Asian states may revisit their relations with China in light of the pandemic.

This book will be of much interest to students of South Asian politics, human security and international relations.

Šumit Ganguly is a Distinguished Professor of Political Science and holds the Tagore Chair in Indian Cultures and Civilizations at Indiana University, Bloomington.

Dinsha Mistree is a Research Fellow in the Program on Strengthening US-India Relations Program at the Hoover Institution and a Research Fellow at Stanford Law School.

Asian Security Studies

Series Editors: Sumit Ganguly, *Indiana University, USA*, Andrew Scobell, *United States Institute of Peace, USA*, and Alice Ba, *University of Delaware, USA*.

Few regions of the world are fraught with as many security questions as Asia. Within this region it is possible to study great power rivalries, irredentist conflicts, nuclear and ballistic missile proliferation, secessionist movements, ethnoreligious conflicts and inter-state wars. This book series publishes the best possible scholarship on the security issues affecting the region, and includes detailed empirical studies, theoretically oriented case studies and policy-relevant analyses as well as more general works.

India's Nuclear Proliferation Policy
The Impact of Secrecy on Decision Making, 1980–2010
Gaurav Kampani

China's Quest for Foreign Technology
Beyond Espionage
Edited by William C. Hannas and Didi Kirsten Tatlow

US-China Foreign Relations
Power Transition and its Implications for Europe and Asia
Edited by Robert S. Ross, Øystein Tunsjø and Wang Dong

Explaining Contemporary Asian Military Modernization
The Myth of Asia's Arms Race
Sheryn Lee

The Covid-19 Crisis in South Asia
Coping with the Pandemic
Edited by Sumit Ganguly and Dinsha Mistree

Chinese Power and Artificial Intelligence
Perspectives and Challenges
Edited by William C. Hannas and Huey-Meei Chang

For more information about this series, please visit: www.routledge.com/Asian-Security-Studies/book-series/ASS

The Covid-19 Crisis in South Asia

Coping with the Pandemic

Edited by
Šumit Ganguly and Dinsha Mistree

Routledge
Taylor & Francis Group

LONDON AND NEW YORK

First published 2022
by Routledge
4 Park Square, Milton Park, Abingdon, Oxon OX14 4RN

and by Routledge
605 Third Avenue, New York, NY 10017

Routledge is an imprint of the Taylor & Francis Group, an informa business

British Library Cataloguing-in-Publication Data
A catalogue record for this book is available from the British Library

Library of Congress Cataloging-in-Publication Data
A catalog record has been requested for this book

ISBN: 978-1-032-16345-1 (hbk)
ISBN: 978-1-032-16346-8 (pbk)
ISBN: 978-1-003-24814-9 (ebk)

DOI: 10.4324/9781003248149

Typeset in Goudy
by Taylor & Francis Books

Contents

Illustrations

Figures

Tables

Contributors

Sumit Ganguly, Rabindranath Tagore Chair in Indian Cultures and Civilizations and Distinguished Professor of Political Science at Indiana University, Bloomington

Dinsha Mistree, Research Fellow at the Hoover Institution and at Stanford Law School

Bipin Adhikari, Researcher at Centre for Tropical Medicine and Global Health, Nuffield Department of Medicine, University of Oxford, Oxford, UK

Rajesh Basrur, Senior Fellow in the South Asia Programme at the S. Rajaratnam School of International Studies at Nanyang Technological University in Singapore

Nicolas Blarel, Associate Professor of International Relations at the Institute of Political Science, Leiden University

Surupa Gupta, Professor of Political Science and International Affairs at University of Mary Washington

Sahar Khan, Research Fellow at the Cato Institute and Adjunct Faculty at the School of Foreign Affairs at American University

Andrea Malji, Assistant Professor in the Department of History and International Studies at Hawaii Pacific University

Shiva Raj Mishra, Research Fellow at The School of Population and Global Health at the University of Melbourne and Nepal Development Society

Karthik Nachiappan, Research Fellow at the Institute of South Asian Studies, National University of Singapore

Ali Riaz, Distinguished Professor in the Department of Politics and Government at Illinois State University

1 Introduction

The Covid-19 Crisis in South Asia: Coping with the Pandemic

Sumit Ganguly and Dinsha Mistree

The ongoing Covid-19 pandemic is the most serious tragedy to afflict South Asia since the end of British colonization. Hundreds of thousands of people have died, and millions more have faced health challenges serious enough to require hospitalization. Apart from the human suffering, the economic toll has been staggering, with economies across the region shutting down for extended periods, to reopen open at partial strength.

Although they were not responsible for the initial outbreak of Covid-19, the five principal states of South Asia—namely Bangladesh, India, Nepal, Pakistan, and Sri Lanka—each had to craft and execute responses to what ultimately became a pandemic. The decisions that were made by the governments of South Asia carried serious consequences, not just for the people of South Asia, but for all people across the world. For example, consider the emergence of the Delta variant of SARS-CoV-2. The Delta variant emerged in India in late 2020. Over the next several months, the Indian government actively downplayed the threat of Covid-19 and encouraged the country to return to normal operations. Scientists and public health officials were discouraged from conducting investigations, and only a chosen few could make public statements. Without much resistance, the Delta variant rapidly spread through India, ultimately overwhelming a country that was not prepared for such a virulent strain of the virus. The Delta variant soon spread to other countries in the rest of the region and across the world, in a disturbing demonstration of the international nature of this pandemic. What could have instead transpired? One need only look at the Omicron variant, which was detected in South Africa in November 2021. Instead of trying to understate the dangers of this new strain, South Africa's own scientists and health officials brought attention to this new variant. Although the Omicron variant is likely to spread through the rest of the world, the freedom of frontline scientists to speak to the new threat—combined with a supportive South African government—has given the rest of the world a chance to contain this new variant and has enabled researchers the opportunity to begin processes much earlier.

This volume assesses how the states of South Asia have so far performed in responding to the Covid-19 pandemic. As of the time of writing (early

DOI: 10.4324/9781003248149-1

2022), the Covid-19 pandemic continued to rage. Scholarship on the political determinants and effects of Covid-19 is scant, and for good reason: it is always easier to assess crises and politics when one knows how the story ends. But the contributors to this volume have commendably chosen to examine the politics of the Covid-19 pandemic to date.

The core proposition of this volume is that politics are playing a central and unwelcome role in how states respond to the Covid-19 pandemic. Across the world—and especially in South Asia—technical guidance and subject matter expertise have frequently been marginalized. Instead of deferring to experts, the pandemic response for most states has been set by politicians, generalist bureaucrats, and even militaries. As a result, processes of policy decision-making and policy execution are often colored by considerations that go beyond public health. Also, with the sidelining of expertise, we see a corresponding neglect in cross-state coordinated pandemic response. If public health officials truly had the power to craft state-level policies, they could rely on transnational epistemic networks to inform and coordinate policy. We contend that the real challenge of managing this pandemic involves getting these processes "right:" if the Covid-19 pandemic is to ever be brought under control, it will require technically informed state intervention with a profound level of international coordination. To get this process of governance right, we must first identify *why* states have marginalized expert-level guidance as they respond to the Covid-19 pandemic, and we must take stock of *how* states are attempting to coordinate pandemic responses on the regional and global stages. Recognizing the possible the risk of a rushed analysis, there is a critical need for scholars to develop a strong understanding of the politics shaping the pandemic response.

Addressing State Capacity

Some might argue that low state capacity is the true culprit limiting an effective pandemic response for the states of South Asia. Owing to decades of chronic underinvestment in public health infrastructure across most of the region, states have long struggled to implement effective public health policy. Consider healthcare spending as a percentage of GDP. For the principal states of South Asia, healthcare spending as a percentage of GDP has been modest: all countries have averaged below 4 percent from 2014 to 2018, with the exception of Nepal (see Table 1.1). For comparison, middle-income countries spent an average of 5.4 percent of their GDP on healthcare in 2018 (World Bank 2021).

Facing limited resources, the states of South Asia have traditionally provided limited basic healthcare services and have instead prioritized addressing and containing disease outbreak. And indeed, we observe that the states of South Asia have a successful track record in dealing with many other instances of infectious disease. Consider India, which coped moderately well when confronted with previous epidemics. For example, despite widespread global

Table 1.1 Healthcare Spending as a Percentage of GDP, 2014–18

Country/Year	2014	2015	2016	2017	2018
Bangladesh	2.5	5.5	2.3	2.3	2.3
India	3.6	3.6	3.5	3.5	3.5
Nepal	5.8	6.2	6.3	5.5	5.8
Pakistan	2.7	2.7	2.9	2.9	3.2
Sri Lanka	3.6	3.9	3.9	3.8	3.8

Source: World Bank. "DataBank: Health, Nutrition, and Population Statistics." World Bank DataBank. Accessed October 8, 2021. https://databank.worldbank.org/source/health-nutrition-and-population-statistics.

concern, India handled the HIV/AIDS crisis of the late 1980s reasonably well. Despite understandable fears, the pandemic did not overwhelm India's public health services. It is possible that public health campaigns, the efforts of various nongovernmental organizations, the rapid development of retroviral drugs, and their production and dissemination across the country stemmed the tide of that particular epidemic. In 1994 there was also a plague outbreak in the western Indian state of Gujarat. Once again, there were reasonable fears that it would sweep across the country. However, a spurt of civic action on the part of many municipalities across the country and the swift distribution of powerful antibiotics contained its spread.

The Covid-19 pandemic, however, has completely overwhelmed India's ramshackle public healthcare apparatus. At first blush, a key difference between the first two epidemics and the current pandemic has to do with the disease vector. HIV/AIDS, as is well known, was based primarily upon sexual transmission. Rudimentary prophylactic measures coupled with a robust information campaign could thereby stem its dispersion. Similarly, the plague outbreak could also be contained with a reasonable effort to tackle waste disposal and the reliance on efficacious antibiotics. In the case of the Covid-19 pandemic, however, given India's population density—especially in major cities where the poor live cheek by jowl—airborne transmission has proven to be highly contagious.

Setting aside differences between the disease vectors, it is also becoming clear that the way in which the Government of India has chosen to respond to the Covid-19 pandemic is different from how it has handled the previous epidemics. At the beginning of the Covid-19 pandemic, government leaders chose to cut off technical expertise from the decision-making process. Prior to the Covid-19 pandemic, India had made considerable investments in building out infectious disease agencies like the National Centre for Disease Control and various structures housed under the Indian Council for Medical Research. According to national-level plans, the leaders of these agencies were supposed to lead and coordinate pandemic response. Instead, these agencies were mostly estranged from the process, with most decisions being routed through the Prime Minister's Office.

What did this decision-making look like for India? As the initial reports of the prevalence of the virus surfaced, in March 2020 the government of Prime Minister Narendra Modi gave four hours' notice before imposing a country-wide lockdown for a duration of three weeks. As all rail, bus, and other modes of public transportation were also shut down, millions of migrant workers were stranded across various parts of the country. In the end, most, but not all of them, wended their way back to their home villages, with some covering several hundred miles on foot. The government, in addition to shutting down most transportation networks, had also made meager economic provisions to assist this acutely vulnerable segment of the country's citizenry.

Even as the Indian government imposed this draconian lockdown, it failed to utilize the breathing space to rapidly acquire personal protection equipment, to boost the capacity of public hospitals, and above all failed to contract public and private firms to swiftly produce vaccines on a mass scale. This particular lapse was especially egregious, as India is no stranger to vaccine production and is, in fact, the largest producer of vaccines in the world. Worse still, apart from state-run facilities, it is also home to the Serum Institute of India, a private company that has long been a producer of vaccines on a mass scale.

Even as the second surge was under way in the early days of 2021, the government's own taskforce on the pandemic did not meet in February or March. Finally, convinced that it had effectively beaten back the virus, the government not only assumed a posture of complacency at home but also went ahead with exporting millions of doses of the vaccine to neighboring countries and beyond as part of an exercise of soft power. In the meanwhile, it failed to stockpile vaccines at home to deal with a possible exigency. Consequently, when the second wave of the virus was well under way, the government was caught completely flatfooted.

Another set of choices on the part of the government led to a significant deterioration in matters. Despite the onset of a second wave of infections, the Bharatiya Janata Party (BJP), faced with elections in four states across India— Assam, Kerala, Tamil Nadu, and West Bengal—and a Union Territory (an administrative unit that reports to New Delhi) decided to proceed with them as planned. Worse still, the Prime Minister and his Minister of Home Affairs, Amit Shah, frequently attended election rallies where no form of social distancing was attempted, let alone practiced, and the vast majority of the attendees were unmasked. To compound matters, the government also permitted the holding of a mammoth Hindu religious festival, the Kumbh Mela, for a period of close to three months starting in January 2021. Over a million devotees participated in this event, where only rudimentary public health measures were implemented to prevent the transmission of the virus.

These lapses alone were shocking enough. However, irresponsible statements from a number of BJP stalwarts did little to advance the cause of public hygiene and medical science. For example, a notable BJP member of parliament (MP) in the state of Uttarakhand claimed that bovine urine was an effective disinfectant and could prevent the spread of the virus. At an election rally in West Bengal another BJP MP claimed that a combination of bovine urine and cold water could eradicate the virus. Finally, although no BJP leader formally endorsed the practice, many people in BJP-ruled states, especially in Gujarat, smeared cow dung on their bodies to ward off the infection. The practice had become so widespread that the head of the Indian Medical Association felt compelled to issue a public notice stating that the procedure had no basis in medical science. Furthermore, it could lead to a false sense of complacency, thereby contributing to increased spread of the virus.

Even after the second wave of infections from Covid-19 engulfed much of the country with public parks being turned into crematoria, bodies being dumped in the Ganga (India's holy river), hospitals running out of spaces to accommodate patients, and some even running out of oxygen, the government directed much of its efforts toward managing the optics of the situation. To that end, it sought to muzzle social media outlets ranging from Facebook to Twitter from posting accounts that highlighted the disastrous conditions prevailing across much of India. And instead of working to forge a national vaccination strategy, in mid-May 2021 it turned over the task to India's states, most of which are ill-equipped, to obtain the necessary vaccines in the first instance.

Apart from India, similar dynamics seem to hold across South Asia. In Sri Lanka and Pakistan, decision-making has been led by the military, whereas Bangladesh's authoritarian leader, Sheikh Hasina, has shown little interest in deferring to experts. Limited implementation capacity has exacerbated the pandemic response, but the fundamental issue concerns the political process of decision-making. Therefore, although we recognize the limitations that states face with respect to implementation capacity in pandemic response, we choose to focus our attention in this volume on the domestic and international politics of pandemic decision-making.

Outline of the Book

This book is divided into two parts. The first part considers domestic responses to the Covid-19 pandemic for the principal states in South Asia. The second part examines how the pandemic is affecting regional engagement. In Chapter 2, Dinsha Mistree empirically compares how the principal states of South Asia have responded to the pandemic. Although these states have all made some correct decisions at certain points in time, no state in South Asia has been able to sustain a successful pandemic response. Mistree argues that the principal states of South Asia have shown an uneven response for three reasons. First, variations in state capacity—and especially in public health capacity—have affected states' abilities to implement effective pandemic responses. Second, policymaking across South Asia has been made with limited—or at least highly selective—technical guidance. Third, populations have not been consistent with respect to complying with safe practices. At the beginning of the Covid-19 pandemic, the public was far more supportive of desirable acts: the public supported and practiced lockdowns, isolation, social distancing, wearing a mask, and so on. As the pandemic has worn on, however, people seem to have grown weary of safe practices.

In Chapter 3, Rajesh Basrur examines how the Covid-19 pandemic is affecting India's quest for status. Basrur cogently describes the struggles and miscalculations that the Indian government made in responding to the pandemic. Basrur suggests that India's failings at addressing the pandemic will ultimately weaken India's standing in the region and in the world.

Chapter 4, by Andrea Malji, considers how the Sri Lanka government has responded to the Covid-19 pandemic. Malji argues that the state's response to the pandemic has been used subversively, to support a larger project of religious marginalization against non-Buddhists. Malji also discusses the success that Sri Lanka had in controlling the virus in the early stages of the pandemic, only to succumb to widespread infection during the second wave.

Sahar Khan considers Pakistan's response to the Covid-19 pandemic in Chapter 5. Reflecting the broader political landscape of Pakistan, Khan describes how the military—rather than the elected civilian government— has been the main decision-maker and executor for enforcing pandemic response policies. The Pakistani military has generally played an outsized role in matters of governance and foreign policy. Khan suggests that the pandemic could reorient the military's focus—and therefore the state's priorities—from a peripatetic foreign policy shaped by great power struggles to a state that focuses on its internal economic needs. Given the numerous weaknesses in the Pakistani economy, such a focus would doubtlessly be welcome by Pakistan's citizens.

In Chapter 6, Shiva Raj Mishra and Bipin Adhikari examine how the state of Nepal has responded to the Covid-19 pandemic. Faced with frequent earthquakes, Nepal is no stranger to crisis management and public health challenges. However, with recent institutional changes, following the adoption of a new constitution in 2015, the pandemic tested these new structures, and particularly the new federal system that has been implemented. On balance, Nepal has performed well in responding to the pandemic—a feat that is especially impressive given the limited resources that the state faces.

The Covid-19 pandemic is also reshaping international relations on the subcontinent. The pandemic has laid bare several new cross-border challenges and opportunities that states will have to contend with in the future. Part 2 of the volume therefore focuses on international relations across South Asia. Chapter 7, by Ali Riaz, examines how India and China have pursued vaccine diplomacy with Bangladesh. The latter initially relied on vaccines from India, rejecting offers for the Chinese Sinovac vaccine. Things changed, however, when India found itself in the throes of the worst stages of the Delta variant. Bangladesh was not able to secure a stable flow of vaccines, and therefore turned to China. For India, mismanagement at home carried pernicious consequences for international actions.[1]

In Chapter 8, Nicolas Blarel takes the human dimension of pandemic-related suffering into account by considering the effects on India's diaspora working in the Gulf states. India has been supplying low-wage, low-skilled labor to the Gulf states for more than two decades. This population of Indian labor-focused migrants working in the Gulf states has proven to be especially vulnerable to the Covid-19 pandemic. The approach of the Gulf states has been to repatriate these migrants in their home countries until the end of the pandemic. Returning such large populations of migrant labor has created an unexpected burden as they must be screened and tracked upon returning to their home countries.

Chapter 9, by Karthik Nachiappan, examines how India's engagement with global governance has been affected by the Covid-19 pandemic. Nachiappan argues that during the pandemic, India has turned to "minilateral" networks, hallmarked by collective discussions between a few countries to tackle specific challenges. Indian leadership also seems to have deepened its penchant for engagement with non-state actors like the Gates Foundation and private companies. Nachiappan convincingly argues that while such engagement is being accelerated by the pandemic, it is not unique to the pandemic: on matters of global governance, this new approach will help India considerably as it wrestles through matters of security, trade, and matters concerning technology.

In Chapter 10, Surupa Gupta concludes by considering whether the pandemic will spur future cooperation between the states of South Asia. Gupta sees the pandemic as a wasted opportunity—particularly for India—in forging deeper cooperation between the principal states. Despite engaging in vaccine diplomacy early on, India could not sustain its efforts for promoting region-wide cooperation and showed little interest in leading any effort to do so. Gupta's argument suggests that India must focus on its domestic challenges first before it will ever be able to play a leading role in regional politics.

Note

1 www.thinkglobalhealth.org/article/pandemic-and-future-indias-foreign-policy.

2 Comparing Responses to the Covid-19 Pandemic

Dinsha Mistree

Perhaps no region of the world has felt the effects of the Covid-19 pandemic as severely as the people and the states of South Asia. As of October 2021, an estimated 37.2 million cases of Covid-19 infections had been confirmed in the region, accompanied by more than 500,000 deaths.[1] These estimates almost certainly belie the true toll of the pandemic, as strained healthcare systems have been unable to treat many otherwise preventable deaths, while states will have to contend with the long-term effects of Covid-19 for decades to come. Apart from the direct health impacts of the pandemic, the economies across the region have also slowed, owing in part to government policies and in part to shifting consumer preferences as customers are less likely to shop in crowded areas. This economic slowdown has put a pause in the amazing poverty reduction trends and considerable economic expansion that South Asia has been enjoying over the past two decades.

The purpose of this chapter is to analyze how the principal states of South Asia—Bangladesh, India, Pakistan, Nepal, and Sri Lanka—have so far responded to the Covid-19 pandemic.[2] The central observation is that no state in the region has been able to sustain an effective pandemic response: no state can should be classified as a 'role model' case. Instead, states have employed different strategies in the fight against Covid-19 at different points in time, resulting in drastically different outcomes over time.

As the data in this chapter will suggest, and as other chapters in this volume show more definitively, there seems to be three overarching reasons why state responses have been so uneven over time. First, as the Introductory chapter highlights, variations in state capacity—and especially in public health capacity—have affected states' abilities to implement effective pandemic responses. In localities where a state is absent or under-resourced, it becomes difficult to identify on-the-ground situations, to enforce protection measures, to deliver potentially lifesaving services for those who are infected, or to run coordinated vaccination campaigns. Such shortcomings inevitably complicate efforts to deliver an effective response to the pandemic. But even states with moderate levels of state capacity have failed to utilize that capacity effectively.[3] This suggests a second reason explaining poor performance in response to the pandemic: during this time period, policymaking across these principal states

DOI: 10.4324/9781003248149-2

has mostly suffered from a lack of technical guidance. With some exceptions, politicians, generalist bureaucrats, and military officers have generally made decisions without seriously engaging public health experts. This lack of expert consultation seems to have only worsened as the pandemic continued. Third, populations have shown varying levels of willingness to comply with government directives. Even though the region has on balance displayed relatively high levels of compliance at the beginning of the pandemic, much of the public in these regions have abandoned individual practices that could reduce the spread of the disease. As the pandemic has dragged on, it seems to have become more difficult to reimpose lockdowns or to encourage other safe practices. Just as critically, as this chapter shall suggest, variations in vaccination between countries are due partly to the willingness of people to be vaccinated. Although in some countries—like India—access to vaccines has been the key impediment to uptake, in other countries—like Pakistan—widespread vaccine skepticism has been a major limiting factor.

The remainder of this chapter is structured as follows. In the next section, I present the status of Covid-19 cases, deaths, and vaccinations across the five principal states. Although some states managed to control Covid-19 in the first stage of the pandemic, all five states have been overwhelmed by the Delta variant. Compared to other strains of the coronavirus, the Delta variant seems to be more contagious and more dangerous, especially for younger populations.[4] In the second section, I explore why some states initially managed to mount an effective resistance whereas others failed to do so. In the third section, I consider state performance following the emergence of the Delta variant. Although the virulent nature of the Delta variant itself is responsible for much of the devastation that took place, even the states that had been overseeing effective policies suddenly found it more difficult to implement policy. The fourth section concludes with a discussion of the main factors affecting the performance of the principal states in responding to the Covid-19 pandemic.

1 Patterns of Cases, Deaths, and Vaccinations

Data about the effects of the Covid-19 pandemic should be approached with a healthy degree of skepticism. By this point, enough reports have emerged from across South Asia suggesting that data manipulation is widespread.[5] Nevertheless, even the official projections suggest that Covid-19 has come with considerable time-varying effects. These effects are summarized in Table 2.1. The rates of cases and deaths suggest that for all states in South Asia, the pandemic can be divided into two stages: before and after the onset of the Delta variant. Most countries in South Asia did not seem to realize the dangerous effects of this variant until February. Soon after, the other principal states of South Asia also reported new waves of infections and deaths.

The data suggest that none of the principal states in South Asia has managed to sustain an effective pandemic response. In the first stage of the pandemic,

Table 2.1 COVID-19's Effects in the Principal States of South Asia

	As at February 1, 2021 (Pre-Delta variant)		As at September 28, 2021 (Pre- and Post-Delta variant)		
	Cases per million	Deaths per million	Cases per million	Deaths per million	Fully vaccinated per hundred
Bangladesh	3,221	48.9	9,344	165.2	9.98
India	7,727	110.9	24,197	321.3	16.61
Nepal	9,136	68.4	26,732	374.6	20.91
Pakistan	2,432	52.2	5,521	123.0	12.17
Sri Lanka	3,023	15.0	23,981	594.8	54.25

Source: *Our World in Data COVID-19 Dataset* (2021)

countries like Sri Lanka and Nepal executed mostly strong and effective pandemic responses compared to their South Asian peer countries. Sri Lanka, for instance, was mostly able to control the pandemic through a rigorous system of testing, targeted lockdowns, and contact tracing, with the military filling in for any gaps in more traditional state capacity. Because of these kinds of targeted strategies, Sri Lanka minimized restrictions and was able to keep the country mostly open for most of the second half of 2020. Through February 1, 2021 Sri Lanka had among the lowest number of cases and deaths per million for the region, even while maintaining an aggressive testing regime.

With the emergence of the Delta variant, however, Sri Lanka suffered catastrophically. In response to this new challenge, the Sri Lankan government sought to reintroduce aggressive restrictions, but struggled to do so. From February 1, 2021 until the time of writing (late September 2021) Sri Lanka went from 3,023 reported cases per million to 23,981 reported cases per million, leading to a gut-wrenching near forty-fold increase in the number of deaths per million people. As a result of the Delta variant wave—and the country's inability to mount an effective response—Sri Lanka has suffered more Covid-19 deaths per million people than any of the principal states in South Asia.

Other states have faced a more constant struggle, both before and after the emergence of the Delta variant. India is one such state. Although some regions of India managed more effective responses to the pandemic than others, all corners of the country suffered from a poorly planned and poorly executed response to the pandemic. A bad situation only got worse following the spread of the Delta variant, with official case and death rates soaring in the months that followed. Furthermore, India's reported cases of—and deaths as a result of—Covid-19 are considerable, but few believe the reported numbers match reality. In an article written in July 2021, Anand, Sandefur, and Subramanian challenge the official figure of approximately 400,000 deaths reported by the government.[6] Looking at data from three different sources, Anand et al. conclude that all-cause excess mortality during the pandemic is probably at least an order of magnitude higher than the official estimates. Other on-the-ground reports from crematoria suggest that official state-level numbers were grossly reduced during the peak of the Delta variant wave.[7]

Taken together, a clear trend across all five of the principal states of South Asia can be seen. Although some countries were able to mount relatively successful initial resistance to the pandemic, all countries suffered in the face of the Delta variant. In the next two sections, we consider how the principal states of South Asia responded to the pandemic prior to the emergence of the Delta variant (section 2) and following the emergence of the Delta variant (section 3).

2 Pandemic Response Prior to the Delta Variant (January 2020–February 2021)

The principal states of South Asia generally started implementing protective measures for containing the spread of Covid-19 in January 2020, followed by strict lockdowns in March 2020. The announcement of these initial measures can be observed in Figure 2.1, which shows trends reported by the Oxford COVID-19 Government Response Stringency Index (the "Stringency Index").[8] The Stringency Index tracks daily national-level government policies since the onset of the pandemic. The Stringency Index has been

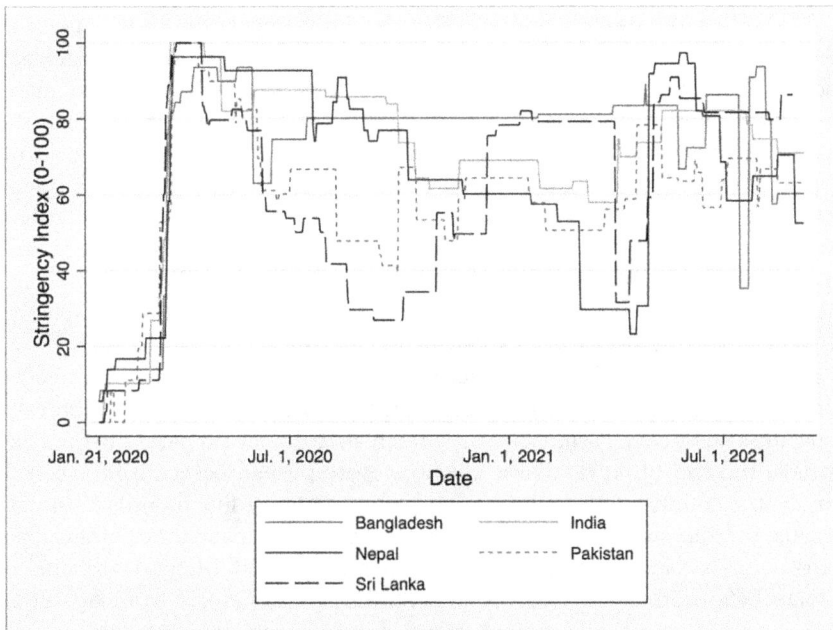

Figure 2.1 South Asia's Government Response Stringency Index
Source: Oxford COVID-19 Government Response Stringency Index

created by scoring government policy decisions across nine indicators: (1) whether the government required schools to close; (2) whether workplace were forced to close; (3) whether public events were canceled; (4) whether there were restrictions placed on the size of allowable gatherings; (5) whether public transport was suspended or not; (6) whether various stay-at-home requirements were adopted; (7–8) whether restrictions were placed on domestic and/or international travel; and (9) whether the government has pursued public information campaigns regarding Covid-19. It should be noted that this Index focuses on policy directives, not on broader policy execution measures or state capacity.

The figure shows that all five principal states of South Asia announced nationwide lockdowns in mid-March 2020, in effect shutting down businesses, schools, and other aspects of society in each country's bid to stanch the spread of the disease. The sudden announcement of nationwide lockdowns was particularly hard for low-wage laborers in India. The government took the decision to shut down the country without considering the downstream consequences of an economic freeze. This lack of contingency planning precipitated a dangerous—and probably avoidable—crisis. Migrant workers suddenly found themselves without jobs, without local safety nets, and few ways to get to their homes, owing to corresponding transportation shutdowns.[9] Even though the country had surplus food, owing to generous farm subsidies, governmental food distribution channels were quickly overwhelmed.

India maintained restrictive lockdown policies from March 25 through June 1, 2020. Over the next several months, the government sought to unlock in phases, but kept many restrictions in place, staying above 60 in the Stringency Index. In contrast, countries like Sri Lanka and Pakistan soon lifted many restrictions after their initial lockdown phases. In the case of Sri Lanka, the lightening of restrictions did not meaningfully increase Covid-19 transmission. Owing to rigorous testing and an effective contact-tracing program, the daily number of Covid-19 cases from June 4 to July 9 never went above 25. On July 10, because of contact tracing, Sri Lanka discovered a Covid-19 outbreak in a prison and was able to isolate the affected population. Also, unlike some other countries that stranded their citizens who lived abroad, Sri Lanka was also able to repatriate more than 54,000 of its citizens by mid-October.[10]

It should be noted that these successes in Sri Lanka were accompanied by serious threats to political freedom and civil liberties. President Gotayaba Rajapaksa dissolved Parliament on March 3, 2020, in preparation for elections at the end of April. These elections were pushed back until August 5, leaving the country with no legislative body for almost five months.[11] In part because of the successful response to the Covid-19 pandemic, Gotayaba's party won parliamentary elections in a landslide, and Mahinda Rajapaksa (Gotayaba's brother) secured the prime ministership. Apart from operating without a branch of government, the person who was put in charge of the country's Covid-19 response, General Shavendra Silva, is banned from entering the United States, as a result of allegedly overseeing unlawful wartime killings at the end of the country's civil war.[12] In addition, the police and the military used the pretense of Covid-19 restrictions to commit several human rights violations.[13] On balance, Sri Lanka's deployment of its military forces to combat the Covid-19 pandemic bolstered state capacity, but also came with threats to civil rights.

Like Sri Lanka, the Pakistani government eased lockdown measures during the summer of 2020. Also like Sri Lanka, Pakistan deployed its military to bolster state capacity in its efforts to contain the spread of Covid-19. The Pakistani army played a central role in acquiring and distributing testing kits, in enforcing localized lockdowns, and in preventing large gatherings. Shortly following the national lockdown, Pakistan organized a National Command and Operation Center to coordinate the state's response to the pandemic. The government also drew on medical experts like Zafar Mirza, a medical doctor who had previously served in the World Health Organization, and Faisal Sultan, an infectious disease expert who had previously been running one of the largest hospitals in the country.

Pakistan also aggressively spent money during the first stage of the pandemic. The government enacted a large-scale cash relief program and declared that frontline healthcare workers who died from the disease would be considered martyrs, providing their families with considerably financial benefits. Toward the end of 2020 the government also began purchasing vaccines, including from China and Russia.

In Bangladesh, the government maintained some of the strongest stringency measures through the summer of 2020, with the final set of restrictions on public movement being lifted on September 1.[14] These measures, however, were mostly maintained on paper, not in practice. Even in April 2020, when almost every other country was able to enforce strict national lockdowns, more than 100,000 Bangladeshis congregated attend a funeral for Maulana Zubayer Ansari attracted more than 100,000 of his supporters.[15] The police were unable to control the crowd, who were mostly unmasked and did not maintain social distancing. Relatedly, the state failed to develop a rigorous testing regimen. Without enough laboratories or test kits, the number of tests conducted per capita ranks the lowest among the five principal states. As a result, it is likely that the number of cases of Covid-19 in Bangladesh have been drastically undercounted.

In Nepal, the government maintained a stringent national lockdown through July 21, 2020. During the national lockdown and afterward, the government of Nepal encouraged the police to issue fines, impound cars, and even detain people who violate government orders regarding curfews, wearing masks, and social distancing. On the whole, however, Nepal's state capacity has proven to be limited, as monitoring and contact tracing could not be scaled up, nor could the country adequately control its borders with India and China, leading to a deluge of incoming cases.[16]

3 Pandemic Response Since the Emergence of the Delta Variant (February 2021–Present)

The Delta variant was first detected in India in October 2020, but did not cause a surge in new cases of infection until mid-February 2021. Because of the central role that India plays in the region, the principal states of South Asia were also exposed to the Delta variant and soon followed India. In response to the wave of cases brought on by the Delta variant, all five of the principal states reimposed protective measures. But as the Stringency Index indicates in Figure 2.1, only two—Nepal and Sri Lanka—reimposed measures along the lines of the initial lockdowns implemented in March and April 2020. Even with these measures, however, the principal states seemed to encounter populations that were unwilling to return to life in lockdown. Even at the height of the Delta variant waves, citizens often refused to practice basic safety measures such as mask wearing and social distancing, let alone observing curfews and lockdowns. A notable exception took place in India, where the carnage of the Delta variant seemed to scare people into compliance.

Nevertheless, the principal states of South Asia have been unable to mount a successful resistance to the Delta variant. For states like Pakistan and Bangladesh, this failure was simply a continuation of the pandemic. In these countries, testing is not widely available and state capacity to enforce pandemic directives is lacking, especially outside of the major cities. Sri Lanka's failure is slightly more puzzling as the state was easily the best in the region at controlling the pandemic prior to the Delta variant. State capacity to enforce pandemic directives seemed strong: there was widespread testing, contact tracing measures were in place, the state had the ability to conduct and enforce localized lockdowns, and so on. But the political will to push strict measures seemed to deteriorate as people had grown weary of the pandemic restrictions. Sri Lanka would temporarily relax measures in April 2021 for the Sinhala and Tamil New Years, a devastating decision that dramatically escalated the number of cases and deaths in the country. By August 2021, Sri Lanka had the fourth-largest daily death totals per capita of any country in the world.[17]

It also bears identifying why India has so far failed to effectively respond to the pandemic. Even though state capacity is weak in certain geographic areas and in certain policy sectors, India has successfully been able to leverage its institutions to respond to prior epidemics.[18] Furthermore, certain states like Kerala have deployed state capacity effectively in its response to the pandemic.[19] The failure to coordinate an effective response to the pandemic is probably due to the nature of policymaking in Delhi. At the outset of the pandemic, the Indian government possessed a world-class system for tracking infectious disease outbreaks in the Integrated Disease Surveillance Programme based at the National Centre for Disease Control. Early into the pandemic, political actors shuttered this program in order to control the numbers of reported cases. Instead, case and death tallies would be issued by the Ministry of Health and Family Welfare. Almost all other major decisions of pandemic response have come out of the Prime Minister's Office, with a coterie of generalist bureaucrats who run various Covid-19 response committees. As with many other policy domains during Modi's tenure, the politicians and generalist bureaucrats who are formulating policy seem to neglect taking expert-level guidance into consideration, even when it is available.[20]

India's failure to coordinate an effective Covid-19 response is perhaps most acute where vaccines are concerned. At the time of writing, only 16.61 percent of the country had been fully vaccinated (see Table 2.1). Given that India is one of the largest global producers of vaccines and prior large-scale vaccination drives have proven successful, one has to wonder why India has struggled to vaccinate.

One would have expected the government to buy vaccines from private producers and then rely on already-existing vaccination distribution mechanisms. However, instead of agreeing to subsidize the costs of vaccine manufacturing, the government encouraged the manufacturers to first sell the vaccines on the private market, with the idea that the proceeds from such sales could then be used to subsidize the supply of lower-cost vaccines. This risky strategy backfired with the outbreak of the Delta variant, when citizens rightly questioned why India was exporting and selling vaccines instead of prioritizing other Indians. The Indian government failed in several other dimensions regarding vaccine procurement and distribution as well, from struggling to help domestic producers source raw materials for the vaccines to refusing to accept donated vaccines produced by Pfizer and Moderna.[21] Not surprisingly, Indian government officials have sought to transfer the blame for low vaccination rates to other actors. During the peak of the pandemic, government officials blamed the United States for dominating the raw ingredient supply chains required to manufacture vaccines.

Government officials have also blamed Indian citizens for low vaccination rates, claiming that misinformation and vaccine hesitancy have hampered vaccination efforts. There is reason to doubt such claims. Indian citizens have historically displayed high levels of confidence in vaccines. In surveys run by the Vaccine Confidence Project between 2015 and 2018, India (along with Bangladesh) ranked among the top countries in the world for vaccine confidence. Additionally, in two non-representative surveys conducted among young adults spread across northern India in May and in July 2021, access to vaccines—rather than vaccine hesitancy—seemed to be the overwhelming challenge.[22] In May 13,579 young adults were asked about whether they were interested in getting vaccinated. Only 5.2 percent (702 respondents) stated that they would not get the vaccine when it became available. By July a separate cohort of 6,060 young adults took a second survey designed to confirm that vaccine hesitancy was not a problem. 98 percent of respondents indicated that they believed vaccines in general are safe (5,631 thought they were very important, 283 somewhat important, 43 not very important, and 87 not at all important). The trend was almost identical for the Covid-19 vaccine specifically, with about 98 percent also stating that this vaccine is important. More than 92 percent of the sample said that they would get a vaccination when it becomes available to them.

Vaccine hesitancy seems to have presented a more serious problem for Pakistan. Prior to the pandemic, Pakistanis have historically grappled with vaccine misinformation and tend to be less confident in vaccines than their counterparts in South Asia.[23] The Pakistani government made a strong push to acquire vaccines for its citizens, turning to China, Russia, the United Kingdom, the United States, and even India. By June 2021 regional governments in Punjab and Sindh were concerned with vaccine hesitancy. Apart from large-scale publicity campaigns and threatening to stop paying government workers who did not get vaccinated, the governments in the two provinces also announced that those refusing vaccinations would lose cellphone service.[24] The threat of such strictures encouraged many Pakistanis to get vaccinated, although Pakistan is now facing the challenge of counterfeit vaccination certificates.[25]

Of the principal states in South Asia, only Sri Lanka has managed to fully vaccinate a majority of its population so far (see Table 2.1). The other countries trail considerably, with Nepal enjoying the next highest vaccination rate at about 20 percent, followed by India at 16 percent. Pakistan and Bangladesh are at 12 percent and 10 percent, respectively. States are struggling to manufacture/acquire vaccines, to distribute them, and to convince reticent citizens to get vaccinated.

Currently, the principal states of South Asia are once again dropping on the Stringency Index. Across the region, schools are reopening, and workers are returning to their jobs. People are once again turning to mass transit systems. Although there is no way of definitively measuring it, people in many parts of South Asia are neglecting to wear masks or to observe social distancing protocols. Observers suggest that people across the region have grown weary of these strictures and are willing to risk their lives if it means a return to normalcy. They no longer believe that their states can protect them.

4 What Went Wrong?

The five principal states of South Asia—Bangladesh, India, Nepal, Pakistan, and Sri Lanka—have all failed to sustain an effective response to the Covid-19 pandemic. Despite all starting with strong national lockdowns, only Sri Lanka (and to a lesser extent, Nepal) were able to effectively protect their citizens from Covid-19 during the first stage of the pandemic. Following the Delta variant, Sri Lanka and Nepal have also struggled to effectively respond to the Covid-19 pandemic, although Sri Lanka deserves praise for its vaccination efforts. What has gone wrong in South Asia?

Scholars generally agree that state performance over a given task is affected by three aspects: (1) the organizational capability of the state to perform a task (i.e., the implementation capability); (2) the political deployment required to effectively respond to the pandemic (i.e., the political process of priority-setting and decision-making); and (3) non-state factors such as the nature of the challenge that the task is designed to address or the willingness of the people to support state directives.[26] In recent years, scholars have suggested that these first two aspects of state performance should both be included in any understanding of state capacity. Scholars in this camp suggest that state capacity is a composite of the state's ability decide and implement policy. Francis Fukuyama, for instance, defines state capacity as "the ability of states to plan and execute policies and to enforce laws cleanly and transparently."[27] Along these lines, the World Bank's "quality of governance" indicators focus on the process of decision-making along with implementation and legitimacy of the process.

More traditional perspectives of state capacity set aside decision-making and political prioritization as a separate process. Borne from the tradition of understanding the state as a tool for exercising power and exerting control, older definitions of state capacity tend to focus on the organizational capability of the state to achieve assigned tasks. For instance, Migdal defines state capacity as "the ability of state leaders to use the agencies of the state to get people in the society to do what they want them to do."[28] In this more traditional framing, state capacity is a separate concept from the political decision-making process. To formulate an effective response to a challenge like the Covid-19 pandemic, a state needs to not only have the institutional machinery in place to execute policy—what is termed as state capacity in this chapter—but it also needs to have the correct political processes in place to identify and formulate effective policy. "State capacity" is used in this section in a traditional manner, as the 'ability to implement decisions.'

Among the principal states, Sri Lanka prior to the Delta variant displayed considerable state capacity. Healthcare workers could conduct Covid-19 tests and treat patients. Meanwhile, the police and the military worked to enforce lockdowns, conduct contact tracing, and encourage other positive behavior. Other states like Bangladesh and Pakistan simply lacked the state capacity to execute effective responses. State capacity not only varies geographically, but can also vary across government sectors. Nepal's state capacity, despite suffering from a lack of resources, also deserves special commendation. Nepal is the only state among the five where the police continue to punish those who break Covid-19 restrictions. Nepal, of course, suffers from low state capacity in healthcare. Nepal's response to the pandemic has been hampered by the paucity of laboratories that can conduct regular testing and the lack of healthcare facilities that can treat those who are infected.

Apart from state capacity, it is telling to observe how decisions are made in each country. In India, the Prime Minister's Office charts most decisions with inputs from a series of Empowered Groups, which are ad-hoc committees including more than one hundred carefully selected government officials, primarily drawn from the ranks of the Indian Administrative

Service (IAS). Officers in the IAS are mostly generalists. Although a small number of them have specialized training, most are not subject matter experts. IAS officers are granted substantial authority and responsibility from early on in their careers, and they generally rise to senior positions by being capable administrators and by tying themselves to the right politicians and political parties. Subject matter experts are expected to feed their views either through these Empowered Groups or through the Ministry of Health and Family Welfare. These experts are able to focus on some finer points of research and medical treatment, but are underutilized, where it comes to making policy. This estrangement of experts also seems to have happened in Bangladesh over the course of the pandemic. In the remaining three states, it seems as though decision-making still involves substantial consultation with subject matter experts.

Setting aside state capacity and the process of decision-making, the data and observations in this chapter suggest that some driving factors in explaining outcomes may be exogenous to state mechanisms. The emergence of the Delta variant—a more infectious and dangerous strain of the coronavirus—seems to have confounded all of the states in South Asia. Another factor affecting state responses to the pandemic is the general malaise of the people. People want to return to their normal lives and appear less likely to cooperate with state sanctions.

What do these observations mean for the future of South Asia? To put it mildly, the prospects of effective state-led responses to the Covid-19 pandemic in South Asia appear grim. With the exception of Sri Lanka and India, states lack the capacity to effectively coordinate a response to the pandemic. Furthermore, expert-level input has been mostly squeezed out of state decision-making processes. Without proper subject-matter expertise, the politicians, generals, and generalist bureaucrats are unlikely to implement the best strategies or to recognize the externalities that come from some policy decisions. Widespread vaccinations could rapidly improve the situation, but states are struggling to acquire and distribute vaccines, including in India, a host to some of the world's best vaccine manufacturing facilities. What is more, outside help in the form of international support is likely to be limited in the region as donor countries are still engaged in controlling outbreaks in their own countries. Perhaps South Asia's best hope is that the virus will mutate itself out of existence, disappearing as swiftly and inexplicably as it arrived.

Notes

1 *Our World in Data COVID-Dataset*, 2021. Data compiled as of September 28, 2021 and include estimated totals for Afghanistan, Bangladesh, Bhutan, India, Maldives, Myanmar, Nepal, and Sri Lanka.
2 The cases of Bhutan, Maldives, and Myanmar have been set aside in this chapter. The reasons for their exclusion have to do with population size for Bhutan and Maldives; in the case of Myanmar, the ongoing instability brought on by the coup of 2020 makes for an uneven comparison with the other principal states.

3 A discussion on defining state capacity is presented in Section 5.
4 Ewen Callaway, "Delta Coronavirus Variant: Scientists Brace for Impact," *Nature*, 2021, 595, pp. 17–18.
5 Puja Changoiwala, "Why South Asia's COVID-19 Numbers Are So Low (For Now)," *Quanta Magazine* June 23, 2020. Available online: www.quantamagazine. org/why-south-asias-covid-19-numbers-are-so-low-for-now-20200623 (Last accessed October 8, 2021).
6 Abhishek Anand, Justin Sandefur, and Arvind Subramanian, "Three New Estimates of India's All-Cause Excess Mortality during the COVID-19 Pandemic," *Center for Global Development Working Paper*, July 2021, no. 589. Available online: https:// cgdev.org/sites/default/files/three-new-estimates-indias-all-cause-excess-mortality-dur ing-covid-19-pandemic.pdf (last accessed October 8, 2021).
7 Jeffrey Gettleman, Sameer Yasir, Hari Kumar, and Suhasini Raj, "As Covid-19 Devastates India, Deaths Go Undercounted," *The New York Times*, April 24, 2021. Available online: www.nytimes.com/2021/04/24/world/asia/india-coronavir us-deaths.html (last accessed October 8, 2021).
8 Thomas Hale, Noam Angrist, Rafael Goldszmidt, Beatriz Kira, Anna Petherick, Toby Phillips, Samuel Webster, Emily Cameron-Blake, Laura Hallas, Saptarshi Majumdar, and Helen Tatlow. (2021). "A Global Panel Database of Pandemic Policies (Oxford COVID-19 Government Response Tracker)." *Nature Human Behavior*, 2021, 5, pp. 529–538.
9 Sumit Ganguly, "India's Coronavirus Pandemic Shines a Light on the Curse of Caste," *The Conversation*, June 2020. Available online. https://theconversation. com/indias-coronavirus-pandemic-shines-a-light-on-the-curse-of-caste-139550.
10 Bilesha Weeratne, "COVID-19 and Migrant Workers: The Economics of Repatria-tion," *Talking Economics Blog*, December 16, 2020. Available online: www.ips.lk/ta lkingeconomics/2020/12/16/covid-19-and-migrant-workers-the-economics-of-repatria tion (last accessed: October 8, 2021).
11 https://www.dw.com/en/coronavirus-keeps-sri-lanka-without-a-functioning-parliam ent/a-53615108.
12 https://www.hrw.org/news/2021/08/06/sri-lanka-police-abuses-surge-amid-covid-19-pa ndemic#.
13 Ibid.
14 Tuhin Adhikary and Wasim Bin Habib, "Curbs on Public Movement Go," *The Daily Star*, Sep. 1, 2020. Available online: www.thedailystar.net/frontpage/news/ curbs-public-movement-go-1953769 (last accessed: October 8, 2021).
15 Abir Mahmud, "100,000 Gather for Funeral in Bangladesh, Defying Lockdown and Sparking Outbreak Fears," CNN.com, Apr. 20, 2020. Available online: https://edi tion.cnn.com/2020/04/19/world/bangladesh-funeral-cornavirus/index.html (Last acces-sed: October 8, 2021).
16 Kusum Sharma, Amrit Banstola, and Rishi Ram Parajuli, "Assessment of COVID-19 Pandemic in Nepal: A Lockdown Scenario Analysis," *Frontiers in Public Health*, 2021, 9: 599280.
17 EconomyNext, "Sri Lanka Records World's Fourth Highest Daily Deaths by Population Amid Lockdown Calls," August 15, 2021. Available online: https:// economynext.com/sri-lanka-records-worlds-fourth-highest-daily-deaths-by-popula tion-amid-lockdown-calls-84902 (last accessed: October 8, 2021).
18 Sumit Ganguly, "Mangling the COVID Crisis: India's Response to the Pandemic," *The Washington Quarterly*, 43, 4, pp. 105–120.
19 Sumit Ganguly and Dinsha Mistree, "Fragile India, Strong India," *Foreign Policy*, May 28, 2021. Available online: https://foreignpolicy.com/2021/05/28/fragile-india -strong-india/ (Last accessed: Oct. 8, 2021).
20 Dinsha Mistree, Rehana Mohammed, and Naman Shah, "The Indian Government's Response to the COVID-19 Pandemic: A Case of Experts in Estrangement," 2021.

21 At the time of this writing, Indian regulatory authorities have not yet approved the Pfizer or Moderna vaccines, even though millions of donated doses are pending approval.

22 The surveys were conducted among students and employees of Freedom Employability Academy (FEA), which provides free employment skills training to young adults across northern India. The intended purpose of the surveys was to identify prevailing views of vaccine hesitancy in order to design special lessons that would encourage vaccination adoption. However, as the surveys revealed that vaccine hesitancy was so rare, FEA decided no special lesson was necessary. Contact the author for more information about the surveys.

23 Vaccine Confidence Project.

24 Zia ur-Rehman, "Unvaccinated in Pakistan? You Might You're your Cellphone Service," *The New York Times*, June 15, 2021. Available online: www.nytimes.com/2021/06/15/world/pakistan-vaccine-cellphones.html (last accessed: October 9, 2021).

25 Niha Dagia, "Pakistan's Fake Vaccine Certificates," *The Diplomat*, September 29, 2021. Available online: https://thediplomat.com/2021/09/pakistans-fake-vaccine-certificates/ (last accessed October 9, 2021).

26 Miguel Centeno, Atul Kohli, and Deborah Yashar, "Unpacking States in the Developing World: Capacity, Performance, and Politics," in *States in the Developing World*, Miguel Centeno, Atul Kohli, and Deborah Yashar (ed.), 2016 (New York: Cambridge University Press).

27 Francis Fukuyama, *State-Building: Governance and World Order in the 21st Century*, 2004 (Ithaca: Cornell University Press), p. 7.

28 Joel Migdal, *State in Society: Studying How States and Societies Transform and Constitute One Another*, 2001 (New York: Cambridge University Press), p. xiii.

3 India and the Covid-19 Pandemic: the Status Dimension

Rajesh Basrur

The outbreak of the Covid-19 pandemic has been dramatically transformational in many ways. In this chapter, I focus on how it has impacted on India's status or international standing in global politics. India's initial performance was encouraging and seemed to set it on a rising trajectory in terms of both its domestic policy response and its assumption of an international leadership role. However, both aspects received a severe setback as the pandemic eventually hit India hard, exposing glaring weaknesses in its health governance and forcing it to moderate its efforts to project itself as a global savior.[1] The reversal appeared to have left India struggling to keep up even as China, much reviled as the source of the pandemic, forged ahead as a leading player in mitigating the global response to it. However, the concept of status is rather more complex then commonly understood and the response to Covid-19 is only one aspect of it. Besides, India retains a significant status profile in other ways that give it at least the potential—by no means the certainty—of retaining its relatively high international status despite its uneven performance in response to the pandemic.

My central argument is as follows. Though India's ambitious launch of a strategy to raise its status in the context of the Covid-19 pandemic ran into considerable difficulty, its overall performance in status terms has been less catastrophic than might first appear. There are two reasons to consider the serious setback of the autumn of 2020 as a speed bump, albeit a painful one, rather than a catastrophe (to reiterate, I say this explicitly in the context of its quest for higher status). First, its hard power position remains significant in terms of its material attributes and its relationships with its adversaries as well as its friends/partners. And second, its soft power as a leading source of succor in the global response to the pandemic shows signs of recovery at the time of writing (late 2021), while its overall position vis-à-vis China in their status competition remains largely intact despite China's much better counter-Covid-19 performance. In short, the pandemic might have been a setback, but it is arguably a temporary one.

The chapter is organized as follows. First, it reviews the concept of status, paying close attention to its hard and soft power components. It then assesses the impact of the Covid-19 pandemic on global politics generally and on

DOI: 10.4324/9781003248149-3

status specifically. It goes on to examine India's performance at some length with respect to the hard power or material dimension of status: its economic and military capacities and its interactions with other major players. Finally, the chapter focuses on the soft power dimension by reviewing two aspects of India's response to the status challenges of the pandemic: its putative leadership role as a major source of the world's preventive and palliative responses to Covid-19, and, more narrowly, its performance with respect to India-China status competition in the war against the coronavirus. The concluding section argues that, though somewhat bruised and battered, India still shows prospects of attaining enhanced status.

Status and Covid-19

India's status in relation to the pandemic parallels its experience in combating Covid-19. The early months of the pandemic left India relatively less affected and hence in a position to claim a major role in global efforts to counter the virus, but this was relatively short-lived. On April 1, 2020, the death toll per million (seven-day rolling average) for India was less than 0.01. By September 19, it had risen considerably to 0.84, but subsided to a low point of 0.07 on February 7, 2021. Thereafter, there was a dramatic increase in the fatality curve, which peaked at 3.01 on May 17 before declining to 0.38 on July 19. At the time of writing, the figure is 0.22 for September 24, 2021.[2] The sheer size of the country and the large aggregate numbers in cases and deaths was partly responsible for the public perception that India was performing really badly: in late December 2020, India was the second-highest on the list of cumulative infections with 10.2 million cases behind only the United States.[3] But even at that time, of the top 20 countries listed by accumulated cases, India ranked 19th in terms of deaths per million with 107 and stood 43rd among the top 50 states in the same list.[4]

Against this, there is evidence that the actual number of cases and fatalities in India has been much higher than the official figures given out by the Indian state, though this is also true of many other states.[5] Still, my main point is that the image of India as a state characterized by incompetent governance—while substantially true—was somewhat distorted in a world where similar incompetence, plus other factors such as the impact of mutations in the Covid-19 virus and public resistance to tight controls, was widespread. The overall effect was to generate significant ups and downs in the image of India, once seen as a rising power, but now presenting an image of failure by hitting the headlines with news of its rising cases and fatalities. As will be seen, the status effects on India have been less severe than they appeared.

Before we come to that, let me first clarify what I mean by status as a concept in the present context. The term has drawn considerable interest in recent work on international politics.[6] It has also been analyzed in an increasingly nuanced way in contrast with the conventional notion that status is a direct derivative of power.[7] Status is defined here as 'filling a place in a social hierarchy' which connotes rank, prestige and, usually, a positive image.[8] Historically, high status has largely been equated with the possession of material power, but that is no longer the case and considerable attention has been devoted to its normative or ideational aspect, sometimes linked with 'soft power'.[9] While hard power, chiefly military and economic, remains the primary currency of international status, non-material aspects of hard power—notably, what one does with it (for instance, its responsible usage)—and other factors such as the image that goes with promotion of the public good and with good domestic governance are important additional sources of status. For instance, the practice of democracy is considered a marker of high status.[10]

Independent India has been considerably preoccupied with status seeking.[11] While much has been made of India as a rising power, some have expressed reservations, arguing that India needs to pull its socks up with respect to domestic governance or that India's potential to shape the world has been exaggerated.[12] From a critic's standpoint, India's poorly developed health infrastructure and inadequate policy response have produced an erratic performance vis-à-vis the pandemic and checked its claims to leadership. This has put India in a difficult position even as the rapid spread of Covid-19 has intensified geopolitical competition, an unsurprising development given the historical linkage between pandemics and global order.[13]

In this chapter, I examine the two dimensions of status separately. The next section examines the impact of the pandemic on India's hard power position. Drawing on the analytical framework developed by Basrur and Sullivan de Estrada, I explore the economic and military-strategic effects of the pandemic, but within a comparative perspective that bears in mind the status effects of other developments in a world order in flux. The subsequent section investigates India's uneven efforts—shaped by the course of the pandemic—to project itself as a leading player in global counter-Covid-19 efforts both in a general sense and in competition with China.

Hard Power Effects on India's Status

Economic Effects

Prime Minister Narendra Modi's imposition of a nation-wide lockdown in March 2020 had acutely negative immediate consequences as productive activity virtually ground to a halt. According to Organization for Economic Cooperation and Development estimates, India's gross domestic product (GDP) contracted by 9.9 percent in 2020.[14] The Modi government's response was meagre in terms of the financial rescue needed to alleviate the hardships of the poorer sections of Indian society. As a Bloomberg report pointed out, the relief package of US$22.5 billion amounted to less than 1 percent of India's GDP, much lower than was the case in many other countries.[15] The initial impact of the downturn was severe, and many analysts were pessimistic.[16]

By late December 2020 the picture had changed. India's economic performance had begun to revive, and the outlook appeared surprisingly positive. A *Bloomberg Quint* report of December 18, 2020 noted that Credit Suisse had significantly revised its forecast on India's economy, which in its opinion had turned the corner and was projected to grow faster than expected.[17] This was in line with the December 2020 report of the Asian Development Bank, which expected a sharp recovery in India's GDP growth from a contraction of 8.0 percent in 2020 to growth of about 8 percent in 2021, the latter being higher than the 7.7 percent growth projection for China.[18] Another positive indicator was that the flow of foreign direct investment (FDI) into India continued to be high. Between April and September 2020, even as India was experiencing a major recession, inward FDI rose 15 percent (compared with the same period in the preceding year), reaching US\$ 39.9 billion.[19] Importantly, the *World Economic League Tables 2021* released in December 2020 by the London-based Centre for Economics and Business Research forecast a longer-term surge in growth from 2021 onward, catapulting India's GDP from its current sixth position in global ranking to third in 2030.[20]

However, the surge in cases in the spring and summer of 2021 and India's slow vaccine response caused a major drop in growth before a steady recovery. The growth figures (in percentage terms) for five successive quarters beginning in April 2020 and ending in June 2021 read –22.9, –4.39, 5.25, 8.72, and 31.73.[21] While there was still a long way to go, financial markets were responding favorably. For instance, *Nikkei Asia* reported in May 2021 that there was a surge in Indian unicorns—start-up companies with an initial valuation of over \$1 billion.[22] The picture at the time of writing is far from dismal from the standpoint of economic performance considering the buffeting India received in 2020–21. In status terms, while it is too early to be definitive, India's standing as a major economy was clearly recovering by late 2021.

Strategic Effects

The military-strategic dimension of status has three main components: a state's possession of the instruments of military power; a state's position in major institutions pertaining to world order; and how it responds to threats to its security. On all three counts, India's performance has not been lacking.

With regards to India's military power, India retains its position as the fourth (out of 140) ranked military power—measured as the potential for conventional war making—after the United States, Russia, and China in the *Global Firepower Index* for 2021.[23] The Index assesses a state's capabilities on a range of criteria ranging from military force to natural resources, financial factors and geography. While such indices are not exactly the last word (nuclear-armed states, notably, do not go to war among themselves), they nevertheless contribute to perceptions. Other sources place India at a similar level.[24] Despite its pandemic struggles, India has not slipped down the ranking table.

A second criterion for assessing a state's status is its association with other major powers—in effect, membership of major clubs in international politics. Over the past two decades, India has built a series of strategic partnerships with France, Japan, Russia, the United States, and several other states. These have been bilateral (with all of those named above and others), trilateral (India-US-Japan); and quadrilateral (India-US-Japan-Australia). The last-named—the Quadrilateral Security Dialogue (or 'Quad') has been particularly prominent in recent years. All of these partnerships involve a range of strategically significant activities: military exercises, arms transfers, strategic discussions and intelligence sharing, among others.[25] All have seen India play an active role without, however, signing a formal military alliance, which would involve it in joint planning and operations with the military forces of other states. A key determinant of India's reluctance to go beyond strategic partnerships to military alliances is status—a desire to retain strategic autonomy that goes back to the early days after independence and which rests on the self-image that India is an independent pole in world politics.

In addition to strategic alignments, India also continues to play an active role in a number of multilateral organizations at the global level, such as the Group of Twenty major economies (G20) and the United Nations (where it continues to seek permanent membership of the Security Council and to draw considerable support for it) and regional organizations such as the Shanghai Cooperation Organization. India has also begun to play a role in semi-formal groupings designed to restructure the strategic arrangements pertaining to the world economy, particularly with the aim of reducing supply chain dependence on China, which was underlined by the latter's centrality in pandemic-related supply chains. In September 2020 India and Australia came together to build an effort to this end.[26] A month later, the Quad resolved to strive for 'resilient supply chains'.[27] In this context, India's presence in the Quad is a significant marker of its status as a key player in the global system. Overall, it constitutes a vital element of India's networking response to the rise of China generally and the negative consequences of the pandemic more specifically.

A third aspect of status is how states deal with adversaries, especially whether they demonstrate resoluteness in doing so. One strategic side-effect resulting partly from the pandemic has been the worsening of India's border tensions with both China and Pakistan. It is unlikely to be a coincidence that India-China border tensions intensified at precisely the time when China came under growing pressure from the US on account of the 'trade war' initiated by Washington, the Chinese economy showed signs of slowing, and suspicions were expressed by President Donald Trump and other national leaders that China was responsible for the outbreak of the pandemic. Meanwhile, tensions on the Indian-Pakistani border were exacerbated by the regular use of small arms, resulting in periodic casualties of both military personnel and civilians. Amidst the burgeoning pandemic, Pakistani Prime Minister Imran Khan found himself in difficulties owing to his weak governance and his uncertain political base, which rests on the backing of the army. Khan and the army have been under sustained attack from a combined political opposition under the banner of the Pakistan Democratic Movement.

Modi's government has displayed a characteristically tough response on both its troubled borders. With regards to China, India was taken by surprise by the killing of some 20 Indian soldiers in hand-to-hand combat in June 2020.[28] It was also caught with its guard down when China occupied slices of land along the disputed Line of Actual Control separating the two armies. While accurate reliable information is hard to come by, it appears that India's refusal to back down and its retaliatory killing of an unknown number of Chinese troops, and its occupation of some China-claimed territory has left the situation at a stalemate at the time of writing. With respect to Pakistan, heightened tensions are not new and have undergone a fractious phase for some time.[29] The intensity of cross-border firing has increased with the rising pressure imposed by the pandemic. Thus far, Modi has been able to maintain his strongman image by undertaking rapid responses as in earlier incidents along both borders.

On the material side, then, India's status (and Modi's) has not been too seriously affected by the adverse effects of the Covid-19 pandemic. I now turn to India's efforts to attain enhanced status by demonstrating its credentials as a 'good' state and, more narrowly, by competing with China over gains in status.

Ideational-Normative Effects on India's Status

The Good State

India's initial foreign policy response to the health crisis was a structured one. In terms of its immediate needs, it was able to acquire access to vaccines for its large pharmaceutical manufacturing industry through international collaborations and obtain a substantial emergency loan of 50 billion yen on easy terms from Japan. More broadly, Indian policy focused on demonstrating leadership by projecting itself as a good state.[30] In the present context, this would mean acquiring kudos as a major source of research, vaccine supply, and economic alleviation at three levels: its immediate neighborhood (South Asia), its extended neighborhood (the Indian Ocean arc from South Africa to Australia), and the global system.[31]

With respect to South Asia, encompassing Afghanistan, Bangladesh, Bhutan, the Maldives, Nepal, Pakistan and Sri Lanka, and collectively the South Asian Association for Regional Cooperation (SAARC), India proclaimed a 'Neighborhood First' policy aimed at prioritizing its neighbors for assisting with crisis response. It sought to demonstrate its regional leadership as well as to compete with China, which was also proactive in extending medical and economic assistance. The main features of India's role in the region at the time are summarized here:

- Evacuation of pandemic-affected citizens of Bangladesh and the Maldives from Wuhan, China, immediately after the Covid-19 outbreak there;
- Supply of medicines such as paracetamol, hydroxychloroquine and Remdisivir (the latter two not proven effective, but in demand) as well as gloves, masks and ventilators;
- Establishment of a SAARC Covid-19 Emergency Fund: in March 2020, India took the lead in setting up the fund and committed a sum of $10 million, half the expected total, to it;
- The setting up of a SAARC Covid-19 Electronic Exchange Platform (COINEX) to exchange information among regional health care professionals and for online learning;
- Establishment of a communications infrastructure through a WhatsApp contact group and video conferences of health professionals on patient management, testing and disease surveillance;
- Online training and learning for health care personnel;
- Assurance of early supply of vaccines to neighbors, e.g. a Memorandum of Understanding was signed in November 2020 to supply Bangladesh with 30 million doses;
- Joint production of vaccines by the Serum Institute of India (SII) and Beximco Pharmaceuticals, a Bangladeshi firm;
- Assurance of low prices for vaccines;
- Extension of economic aid: a US$ 250 million financial grant and food aid to the Maldives; and a currency swap arrangement worth $US 400 million extended to Sri Lanka in July 2020;
- Provision of doctors and nurses to the Maldives.

The outreach program was not entirely satisfactory. The quantum of money actually contributed to the fund by India to the SAARC fund as of early December 2020 was just $1.89 million.[32] The Fund fell victim to tensions between India and Pakistan and appears to have lost momentum.[33] As one study notes, senior retired government officials at the time expressed reservations about India's performance, particularly in contrast with that of China, which was carrying out a better-organized aid programme.[34] New Delhi did not appear to have a coherent strategy in place and implementation of commitments was sometimes patchy, as with disbursals to the Fund.

In the wider area of the Indian Ocean region, India did not essay a multilateral effort, but focused on bilateral relationships to help states respond to the pandemic. Some significant examples include:

- Research: India and Australia initiated collaboration on research funded by the Australia-funded Australia-India Strategic Research Fund to promote early detection of long-term health consequences of Covid-19. India and Israel began collaborating on systems for rapid testing for the detection of Covid-19 through swab tests as well as non-invasive means relating to breath, saliva, and sound;

- Debt relief: India provided debt service relief to Myanmar to offset the impact of Covid-19 for the period from May to December 2020;
- Welfare assistance: India provided US$ 1 million for the support of Palestinian refugees affected by the pandemic. The aid was channeled through the United Nations Relief and Works Agency for Palestinian Refugees in the Near East;
- Medical assistance: India provided medical help in a variety of forms to the Middle East, for instance sending doctors and other health professionals to Kuwait; and shipping hydroxychloroquine to Israel, Jordan and Oman. The Indian Navy sent medical teams to Mauritius and Comoros to train health professionals in Covid-19 management;
- Repatriation: India assisted several countries in repatriating their citizens in a time of restricted travel. In reverse, a large number of Indian citizens have been brought home, especially from the Middle East and Southeast Asia;

Globally, India positioned itself as a nation committed to the global good and underlined its commitment to international cooperation in a number of ways:

- Early in the crisis, India removed restrictions on the export of ventilators (March 2020) and medicines (April 2020);
- Medicines: Drugs such as paracetamol and hydroxychloroquine were exported to countries around the world, e.g. Bahrain, Brazil, Germany, Israel, Malaysia, Spain, and the United States;
- Vaccine research: India made arrangements for joint research and trials in collaboration with organizations in Russia, the United Kingdom and the United States as well as with the multilateral organization Gavi, the Vaccine Alliance;
- Vaccine supply (export): India positioned itself as a vaccine supplier to the world—a commitment made by Prime Minister Modi to the United Nations General Assembly in September 2020. It pledged US $15 million to Gavi, which obtains and supplies low-cost vaccines to 92 low- and middle-income countries. The Bill and Melinda Gates Foundation entered into a partnership with SII to accelerate the production and delivery of vaccines around the world. In addition, the Indian firm Wockhardt contracted with the UK government to supply vaccines through the former's subsidiary in Wales. India and the other members of the Quad discussed ways of coordinating the distribution of vaccines;
- Vaccine supply (import): A collaboration between SII and Astra Zeneca aimed to ensure large-scale availability of vaccines. Under an Indo-Russian collaboration, India's Dr Reddy's Laboratories and the Russian Direct Investment Fund, a sovereign wealth fund, agreed on the supply of 100 million doses of the Sputnik V vaccine to India;
- Vaccine supply at lower cost: India joined hands with South Africa and proposed to the World Trade Organization that trade-related intellectual property rights pertaining to pharmaceutical drugs be temporarily

waived in order to lower the cost of vaccines, but this met with opposition from a number of developed countries where the major drug producers are located.[35] US support for the waiver in May 2021 seemed to have improved the prospect of a cheaper vaccine.[36]

All of this generated a positive image of India as a global savior. However, as shown at the outset, India's own performance was far from consistent. By March 2021 India's rank in a global index assessing Covid-19 management stood at a dubious 87 out of 102 states evaluated by the Lowy Institute.[37] While policymakers struggled to maintain a coherent domestic approach, India's international reputation sagged.[38] The adverse publicity attending the dramatic rise in cases and fatalities in medical publications as well as in the popular media dealt a blow to India's image.[39]

There are authoritative arguments to the effect that India's performance was not as bad as widely understood if viewed in comparative terms.[40] But perceptions shape status. Besides, what the sudden increase in the caseload and fatalities did do was to deliver a serious blow to India's Covid-19 diplomacy. From being a major exporter of medicines, equipment and vaccines, India now became an importer. A sharp cutback in the export of vaccines under the *Vaccine Maitri* (=Vaccine Friendship) program meant that poor nations depending on Indian supplies were suddenly left stranded. Between January and March 2021, India had exported 64 million doses; but by mid-April the flow had been reduced to a trickle, with only 1.2 million doses sent out.[41] As a result, the COVID-19 Vaccines Global Access (COVAX) program backed by the World Health Organization (WHO) and Gavi for distribution of cheaper vaccines was disrupted, with some 60 low-income countries deprived of adequate supplies. Meantime, India was compelled to order Russian Sputnik vaccines to make up for its own shortfall. Aid flows encompassing oxygen, medicines and vaccines were sourced to some 40 countries, the WHO, Gavi and private donors, with the US alone committing $500 million by mid-May.[42]

The reversal of fortunes left domestic critics upset by the drop in India's status from an aid giver to an aid recipient.[43] But the Indian government continued to assist others to the extent it could. In June 2021 it reversed its ban on the export of the drug Remdisivir—a hollow measure, as WHO research shows that the drug has no anti-viral effects.[44] In July, Prime Minister Modi announced that the Covid Vaccine Intelligent Work (CoWIN) platform—an electronic platform for managing Covid-related infrastructure—would be made available free of cost to the world.[45] On the vaccine front, the prospects of a rapid expansion of capacity improved. In April 2021, the government announced that the production of the indigenous vaccine Covaxin would be multiplied ten-fold by September.[46] And in August 2021 a new DNA-based vaccine—"ZyCoV-D"—was approved for production and for use by younger age groups as well.[47] By late 2021 it appeared that India was once again poised for the role of a major aid giver in the course of time (barring, of course, a fresh reversal of fortunes spurred by an unpredictable virus). Some uncertainty remained. In October 2021 the government announced that it had resumed vaccine supplies to Bangladesh, Myanmar, Nepal, and Iran.[48] However, it was also the case that the rate of vaccination within India was low (at about 30 percent) and the pace showed signs of slowing down significantly.[49]

Competing with China

India's status competition with China has been a long-standing one.[50] The two were roughly at the same level in material power until the 1970s, but China has forged far ahead of India and is now widely considered the 'challenger' and possible successor to US global hegemony. As recently as 1991, when India's economy began to experience accelerated expansion, its GDP of \$270.10 billion was some 70 percent of China's \$383.37 billion. By 2019 the gap had widened substantially and India's GDP at \$2.86 trillion was just 20 percent of China's \$14.28 trillion. Similarly, India's military spending in 1991 at \$8.6 billion was 87 percent of China's, but by 2019 Indian spending at \$71.1 billion had shrunk to a mere 27 percent of China's \$261.1 billion.[51] What irks many Indians is China's belief that India is not really a peer power.[52] The material gap between the two is reason enough from Beijing's standpoint. In particular, China's immense financial strength has given it a leading position in global investment through the Belt and Road Initiative, which it has used as an instrument of influence worldwide. In addition, China has the institutional advantage of being a permanent member of the Security Council and a recognized 'Nuclear Weapons State' under the Nuclear Nonproliferation Treaty—both status markers denied to India.

Unsurprisingly, the two states have engaged in status competition in response to the pandemic.[53] This reflects a more general phenomenon of intensified competitive behavior resulting from the spread of the virus.[54] We have already seen India's effort to cast itself as a leading player in counter-Covid-19 efforts. Similarly, though beginning with the disadvantage of being the geographical source of the pandemic, China has sought to portray itself as a global benefactor through 'Covid diplomacy' by providing medical aid to other states. In part, this is to offset the bad press it has received for its tough attitude vis-à-vis its maritime border disputes in the South and East China Seas.[55] The results have been mixed. On the plus side, China has been able to generate a substantial flow of medicines, protective equipment, ventilators and vaccines to at least 100 countries[56]. On the negative side, suspicions about China's role in the origins of the pandemic persist and there have been questions about the quality of its supplies, particularly with respect to the efficacy of its vaccines.[57]

While India and China have laid claim to playing a vital role for the common good, both have experienced difficulties. India had the initial advantage of a low infection rate, whereas China was hard hit and widely criticized as the source of the virus. Subsequently, India was buffeted by a wave of infections and later a second and bigger tide, which took away the status advantages of being an aid giver and turned it into an aid recipient, while China was one of the few states able to control the spread of the virus and simultaneously become a major aid provider. But China's difficulties with respect to the effectiveness of its vaccines and its lack of transparency in assisting the international community to trace the origins of the virus have cast a shadow over its reputation.[58]

Ultimately, the status competition arising from the effects of and responses to the pandemic have not produced a significant tilt in the image balance between India and China. At the time of writing, India's Covid-19 resilience is showing signs of returning, while China, though doing much better, has still not been able to eradicate the virus or to overcome the distrust it has generated. Both have done much to back their claims to striving for the public good, but both have fallen short in different ways. Both also retain the potential to perform much better or, if the virus mutates in unpleasant ways, worse.

Conclusion

This review of India's response to the Covid-19 pandemic shows that, on the whole, India has fared unevenly with respect to its status objectives. On the material side, it retains a largely unchanged position with respect to its economic prospects as well as its military-strategic position as a rising power. On the ideational-normative side, India has lost much of its luster in its efforts to project itself as a net provider for the common good, but is showing signs of recovering at least some of its old *élan*. Lastly, India's competitive position vis-à-vis China remains stable as neither state has performed sufficiently well to enable it to overshadow the other's standing.

The prestige gained or lost by India in the context of the pandemic has to be viewed in the wider perspective of its image generally. The millennium began with the growing recognition of India as a 'rising power', but also as a democratic one. Latterly, much of the shine with respect to the latter has worn off. The status gained by India's performance as a successful democracy has been open to question as the Indian state has taken on the characteristics of an increasingly illiberal democracy: intolerance, deterioration in the rule of law, and political repression—none of it new, but looming larger in recent years.[59] An indication of the shift is the steep drop in India's position in the Economist Intelligence Unit's Democracy Index from 27th in 2014 to 53rd in 2020.[60] Ultimately, achievements in attaining enhanced status will be determined by how the India story plays out with regard to the full mix: its reputation as a provider of the public good not only globally, but also in the domestic realm. The jury is still out on the balance between them.

Notes

1   Sumit Ganguly, 2020. 'Mangling the COVID Crisis: India's Response to the Pandemic', *Washington Quarterly*, 43, no. 4: 105–120.
2   Our World in Data. n. d. 'Daily New Confirmed Deaths per Million People', https://ourworldindata.org/covid-deaths?country=~IND#country-by-country-data-on-confirmed-deaths (accessed September 28, 2021).
3   Worldometer, 'Reported Cases and Deaths by Country, Territory, or Conveyance'. December 28, 2020, www.worldometers.info/coronavirus/(accessed same day).
4   Ibid.
5   Soutik Biswas, 'Covid-19: India Excess Deaths Cross Four Million, Says Study', BBC News July 20, 2021, www.bbc.com/news/world-asia-india-57888460 (accessed same day).
6   Rajesh Basrur and Kate Sullivan de Estrada, *Rising India: Status and Power* (Abingdon and New York: Routledge, 2017); 'Emel Parlar Dal' 'Status Competition and Rising Powers in Global Governance', *Contemporary Politics*, 25, no. 5 (2019):1–13; Khong Yuen Foong, 'Power as Prestige in World Politics', *International Affairs*, 95, no. 1 (2019): 119–142; T.V. Paul, Deborah Welch Larson, and William C. Wohlforth, eds, *Status in World Politics* (New York: Cambridge University Press, 2014); Thomas J. Volgy, Renato Corbetta, Keith A. Grant, and Ryan G. Baird, eds, *Major Powers and the Quest for Status in International Politics* (New York: Palgrave Macmillan, 2011); Steven Michael Ward, 'Lost in Translation: Social Identity Theory and the Study of Status in World Politics', *International Studies Quarterly*, 61, no. 4 (2017): 821–834.
7   Emel Parlar Dal, 'Status-seeking Policies of Middle Powers in Status Clubs: the Case of Turkey in the G20', *Contemporary Politics*, 25, no. 5 (2019): 586–602; Deborah Welch Larson, 'Status and World Order', in *Status in World Politics*, ed. T.V. Paul, Deborah Welch Larson and William C. Wohlforth (New York: Cambridge University Press, 2014), 3–30; Thomas J. Volgy and Kelly Marie Gordell, 'Rising Powers, Status Competition, and Global Governance: A Closer Look at Three Contested Concepts for Analyzing Status Dynamics', *International Politics*, 25, no. 5 (2018): 512–531.
8   William C. Wohlforth, Benjamin de Carvalho, Halvard Leira and Iver B. Neumann, 'Moral Authority and Status in International Relations: Good States and the Social Dimension of Status Seeking', *Review of International Studies*, 44, no. 3: 526–546 (2017), 528.
9   Matthew Kroenig, Melissa McAdam and Steven Weber, 'Taking Soft Power Seriously,' *Comparative Strategy*, 29, no. 5 (2010): 412–431; Joseph Nye, *Soft Power: The Means to Success in World Politics* (New York: Public Affairs, 2004).
10 Rajesh Basrur and Kate Sullivan de Estrada, *Rising India: Status and Power* (Abingdon and New York: Routledge, 2017), 10–12, 46–8; Deborah Welch Larson, 'Status and World Order', in *Status in World Politics*, ed. T.V. Paul, Deborah Welch Larson and William C. Wohlforth (New York: Cambridge University Press, 2014), 24.
11 Basrur and Sullivan de Estrada, *Rising India: Status and Power*; Baldev Raj Nayar and T.V. Paul, *India in the World Order: Searching for Major Power Status* (Cambridge: Cambridge University Press, 2003); T.V. Paul and Mahesh Shanker, 'Status Accommodation through Institutional Means: India's Rise in the Global Order', in *Status in World Politics*, ed. Paul, Larson, and 165–191.
12 Sumit Ganguly, 'Think Again: India's Rise', *Foreign Policy*, July 5, 2012, https://foreignpolicy.com/2012/07/05/think-again-indias-rise (accessed on September 28, 2021; Amrita Narlikar, 'All that Glitters Is Not Gold: India's Rise to Power', *Third World Quarterly*, 2, no. 5 (2007): 983–996.

13 David P. Fidler, 'The Covid-19 Pandemic, Geopolitics, and International Law,' *Journal of International Humanitarian Legal Studies*, 11, no. 2 (2020): 237–248.

14 Organization for Economic Cooperation and Development, 'A Brighter Outlook But Recovery Will Be Gradual', n.d. www.oecd.org/economic-outlook (accessed on December 28, 2020).

15 Katharina Buchholz, 'Who Is the Indian Government Aid Package Benefiting?' Bloomberg, April 1, 2020, www.statista.com/chart/21308/indian-government-coronavirus-aid-package (accessed same day).

16 Praveen Chakravarty, 'What the Indian Markets Don't Tell You', *Hindustan Times*, November 30, 2020, www.hindustantimes.com/analysis/what-the-indian-markets-don-t-tell-you-analysis/story-j0I63mX5tJ5a5QggToY88J.html (accessed same day); Jeffrey Gettleman, 'Coronavirus Shatters India's Big Dreams', *The New York Times*, September 5, 2020, www.nytimes.com/2020/09/05/world/asia/india-economy-coronavirus.html?campaign_id=2&emc=edit_th_20200905&instance_id=21942&nl=todaysheadlines&regi_id=30381051&segment_id=37504&user_id=fa090cc506ce13db9a05faea5d295a62 (accessed same day); 'Oxford Economics Revises Downwards India Growth Forecast; Pegs at Average 4.5 pc for 2020–25', *Outlook*, November 19, 2020, www.outlookindia.com/newsscroll/oxford-economics-revises-downwards-india-growth-forecast-pegs-at-average-45-pc-for-202025/1978630 (accessed same day).

17 Mahima Kapoor, 'Covid-19 Pandemic's Lasting Cost on Indian Economy Smaller than Expected: Neelkanth Mishra', *Bloomberg Quint*, December 18, 2020, www.bloombergquint.com/economy-finance/pandemics-lasting-cost-on-india n-economy-smaller-than-expected-neelkanth-mishra (accessed same day).

18 Asian Development Bank, *Asian Development Outlook Supplement*, December 2020, p. 7 (Table), www.adb.org/sites/default/files/publication/658721/ado-supplement-december-2020.pdf (accessed same day).

19 Prathamesh Mulye, 'Foreign Investors Poured $39 Billion into India When the Economy Was at Its Worst,' *Quartz India*, December 5, 2020, https://qz.com/india/1941596/fdi-into-india-rose-despite-coronavirus-lockdown-recession/ (accessed on same day).

20 Centre for Economics and Business Research, *World Economic League Table 2021*, December 29, 2020, https://cebr.com/reports/world-economic-league-table-2021/ (accessed on October 19, 2021).

21 'Quarterly GDP Growth of India', *Statistics Times*, September 4, 2021, https://statisticstimes.com/economy/country/india-quarterly-gdp-growth.php. (accessed on September 28, 2021).

22 Wataru Suzuki, 'India Emerges as China's Tech Challenger with Record Unicorn Run', *Nikkei Asia*, May 3, 2021, https://asia.nikkei.com/Spotlight/Market-Spotlight/India-emerges-as-China-s-tech-challenger-with-record-unicorn-run (accessed on same day).

23 *Global Firepower 2021*. GlobalFirepower.com, n.d. [2021], https://www.globalfirepower.com/ (accessed September 28, 2021).

24 Mark Episkopos, 'Ranked for 2021: Top 5 Militaries on Planet Earth,' *National Interest*, February 20, 2021, https://nationalinterest.org/blog/buzz/ranked-2021-top-5-militaries-planet-earth-178555 (accessed September 28, 2021).

25 Rajesh Basrur and Sumitha Narayanan Kutty, 'Modi's India and Japan: Nested Strategic Partnerships,' *International Politics*. February 2021, doi: https://link.springer.com/article/10.1057/s41311-021-00288-2.

26 Kiran Sharma, 'Japan, India and Australia Aim to Steer Supply Chains around China,' Nikkei Asia, September 1, 2020, https://asia.nikkei.com/Economy/Trade/Japan-India-and-Australia-aim-to-steer-supply-chains-around-China (accessed on November 17, 2020).

27 Minister for Foreign Affairs, Australia. 'Australia-India-Japan-United States Quad Foreign Ministers' Meeting', October 6, 2020, www.foreignminister.gov.au/minis

ter/marise-payne/media-release/australia-india-japan-united-states-quad-foreign-minis ters-meeting (accessed on November 17, 2020).

28 Joshi, Manoj. 2021. *Eastern Ladakh: the Longer Perspective*. Observer Research Foundation, New Delhi, June 14. www.orfonline.org/research/eastern-ladakh-the-longer-perspective (accessed same day); Arzan Tarapore, *The Crisis after the Crisis: How Ladakh Will Shape India's Competition with China*. Lowy Institute, Sydney, May 2021, (accessed September 28, 2021).

29 Sushant Singh, 'Guns Fall Silent on the LoC: But Can Peace Follow?' India Forum, March 5, 2021, www.theindiaforum.in/article/guns-fall-silent-loc (accessed on September 28, 2021); John Vater and Yogesh Joshi, *Narendra Modi and the Transformation of India's Pakistan Policy*, Institute of South Asian Studies, National University of Singapore, August 5, 2020, www.isas.nus.edu.sg/papers/narendra-modi-and-the-tra nsformation-of-indias-pakistan-policy (accessed October 19, 2020).

30 Gareth Evans, 'Foreign Policy and Good International Citizenship,' Address by the Minister for Foreign Affairs, Senator Gareth Evans, Canberra, March 6, 1990, www.gevans.org/speeches/old/1990/060390_fm_fpandgoodinternationalcitizen.pdf (accessed on November 26, 2016); Peter Lawler, 'The "Good State" Debate in International Relations', *International Politics*, 50, no. 1 (2013): 18–37.

31 Harsh V. Pant and Anant Singh Mann, *India's Public Health Diplomacy in the Time of Covid19* [sic], Observer Research Foundation, New Delhi, June 13, 2020, www.orfonline.org/expert-speak/indias-public-health-diplomacy-in-the-tim e-of-covid19-67783 (accessed on same day); Smruti S. Pattanaik, 'SAARC COVID-19 Fund: Calibrating a Regional Response to the Pandemic', *Strategic Analysis*, 44, no. 3 (2020): 241–252; Smruti S. Pattanaik, 'COVID-19 Pandemic and India's Regional Diplomacy', *South Asian Survey*, 28, no. 1 (2021): 92–110; Saran, Shyam, Gautam Mukhopadhaya, Nimmi Kurian and Sandeep Bhardwaj. *India as the Engine of Recovery for South Asia: A Multi-sectoral Plan for India's Covid-19 Diplomacy in the Region*, Centre for Policy Research, New Delhi, August 19, 2020, www.cprindia.org/research/reports/india-engine-recovery-south-asia-multi-sectoral-plan-india%E2%80%99s-covid-19-diplomacy-0 (accessed on same day); Sonali Singh, *India's Response to Covid-19: A Soft Power Perspective*, Center on Public Diplomacy, University of Southern California, Los Angeles, May 15, 2020, https://uscpublicdiplomacy.org/blog/india%E2%80%99s-response-covid-19-soft-p ower-perspective (accessed on same day).

32 Author's calculation from Soni Mishra, 'In India's COVID Funds for SAARC Nations, Nepal Gets Lion's Share,' *Week*, December 03, 2020, www.theweek.in/news/india/2020/12/03/in-india-covid-funds-for-saarc-nations-nepal-gets-lion-share.html (accessed October 19, 2021).

33 Pattanaik, 'COVID-19 Pandemic and India's Regional Diplomacy': 104.

34 Shyam Saran, Gautam Mukhopadhaya, Nimmi Kurian and Sandeep Bhardwaj, *India as the Engine of Recovery for South Asia: A Multi-sectoral Plan for India's Covid-19 Diplomacy in the Region*, Centre for Policy Research, New Delhi, August 19, 2020, www.cprindia.org/research/reports/india-engine-recovery-south-asia-multi-sectoral-pla n-india%E2%80%99s-covid-19-diplomacy-0 (accessed on same day).

35 Andrew Green, 'At WTO, a Battle for Access to COVID-19 Vaccines', *Devex*, Washington, DC, December 15, 2020, www.devex.com/news/at-wto-a-battle-for-a ccess-to-covid-19-vaccines-98787 (accessed on same day); Nancy S. Jecker and Caesar A. Atuire, 'What's Yours is Ours: Waiving Intellectual Property Protections for COVID-19 Vaccines', *Journal of Medical Ethics*, 47, no. 9 (2021): 595–98.

36 'Covid: US Backs Waiver on Vaccine Patents to Boost Supply,' BBC News, May 5, 2021, www.bbc.com/news/world-us-canada-57004302 (accessed on September 30, 2021).

37 *Covid Performance Index*. Lowy Institute, Sydney, n.d. [2021] https://interactives. lowyinstitute.org/features/covid-performance (accessed September 28, 2021).

38 Pradeep Taneja and Azad Singh Bali, 'India's Domestic and Foreign Policy Responses to COVID-19', *Round Table*, 110, no. 1 (2021): 46–61.

39 'India's COVID-19 Emergency', *Lancet*, May 8, 2021, www.thelancet.com/journals/lancet/article/PIIS0140-6736(21)01052–7/fulltext (accessed on September 28, 2021); Karan Deep Singh, 'As India's Lethal Covid Wave Neared, Politics Overrode Science', *The New York Times*. September 14, 2021, www.nytimes.com/2021/09/14/world/asia/india-modi-science-icmr.html?campaign_id=2&emc=edit_th_20210914&instance_id=40328&nl=todaysheadlines&regi_id=30381051&segment_id=68851&user_id=fa090cc506ce13db9a05faea5d295a62 (accessed on same day).

40 Dhavendra Kumar and Madhukar Mittal, 'India's COVID-19 Emergency: Overarching Conclusions Belie Facts', *Lancet*, June 26, 2021, www.thelancet.com/journals/lancet/article/PIIS0140-6736(21)01243–5/fulltext (accessed September 29, 2021).

41 Neha Arora and Krishna N. Das, 'Analysis: India Shifts from Mass Vaccine Exporter to Importer, Worrying the World', Reuters, April 16, 2021, www.reuters.com/world/india/india-shifts-mass-vaccine-exporter-importer-worrying-world-2021-04-16 (accessed on same day).

42 'From the US to Bahrain: The Countries that Have Sent Covid Relief Material to India So Far', *Indian Express*, May 1, 2021, https://indianexpress.com/article/india/from-the-us-to-bahrain-the-countries-that-have-sent-covid-relief-material-to-india-so-far-7297967/ (accessed on same day); 'In A Graphic: Global Aid for India's Battle against the Deadly Second Wave', *India Today*, April 29, 2021, www.indiatoday.in/india-today-insight/story/in-a-graphic-global-aid-for-india-s-battle-against-the-deadly-second-wave-1796430-2021-04-29 (accessed on same day); *Tribune*, 2021. 'US Has Provided over USD 500 Million in COVID Relief to India, Says White House', *Tribune*, May 20, 2021, www.tribuneindia.com/news/nation/us-has-provided-over-usd-500-million-in-covid-relief-to-india-says-white-house-255753 (accessed on same day).

43 Manjari Chatterjee Miller and Vidhu Priya Mukundan, 'The Politics of Foreign Aid in India', *Hindustan Times*, June 20, 2021, www.hindustantimes.com/opinion/the-politics-of-foreign-aid-in-india-101624200153853.html (accessed on same day).

44 'Remdesivir, HCQ Have No Antiviral Effects: WHO Study', *Statesman*, July 13, 2021, www.thestatesman.com/world/remdesivir-hcq-no-antiviral-effects-study-1502981560.html (accessed on same day).

45 Geeta Mohan, 'India's CoWIN Platform Is Now Open-source to Help World Combat Covid-19: PM Modi', *India Today*, July 5, 2021, www.indiatoday.in/coronavirus-outbreak/story/cowin-global-conclave-2021-pm-modi-speech-open-source-1824208-2021-07-05 (accessed on same day).

46 'Covaxin Production to Increase 10 Times by September 2021: Union Minister Harsh Vardhan', *New Indian Express*, April 8, 2021, www.newindianexpress.com/nation/2021/apr/18/covaxin-production-to-increase-10-times-by-september-2021-union-minister-harsh-vardhan-2291641.html (accessed September 29, 2021).

47 'Zydus Cadila: What We Know about India's New Covid Vaccines', BBC News, August 23, 2021, www.bbc.com/news/world-asia-india-55748124 (accessed on September 29, 2021); Smriti Mallapaty, 'India's DNA COVID Vaccine Is A World First – More Are Coming', *Nature*, September 2, 2021, www.nature.com/articles/d41586-021-02385-x (accessed on September 26, 2021).

48 'India Resumes Vaccine Exports to Neighbours,' *Tribune*, October 15, 2021, www.tribuneindia.com/news/nation/india-resumes-vaccine-export-to-neighbours-324750 (accessed on same day).

49 'India's Covid Vaccination Campaign Slows Down Despite Record Production', *Telegraph*, October 18, 2021 www.telegraphindia.com/india/indias-covid-vaccination-campaign-slows-down-despite-record-production/cid/1834966 (accessed on same day).

50 David Brewster, 'India and China at Sea: A Contest of Status and Legitimacy in the Indian Ocean', *Asia Policy*, 22 (2016): 4–10; Deborah Welch Larson, 'Status Competition among Russia, India, and China in Clubs: A Source of Stalemate or Innovation in Global Governance', *Contemporary Politics*, 25, no. 5 (2019): 549–66; Kate Sullivan de Estrada and Rosemary Foot, 'China's and India's Search for International Status through the UN System: Competition and Complementarity', *Contemporary Politics*, 25, no. 5 (2019): 567–85.

51 Author's calculations based on data from World Bank, n.d., 'GDP Growth (Annual %) – India', https://data.worldbank.org/indicator/NY.GDP.MKTP.KD. ZG?end=2019&locations=IN&start=1991&year_low_desc=true (accessed on May 22, 2021).

52 Manjeet S. Pardesi, 'Explaining the Asymmetry in the Sino-Indian Strategic Rivalry', *Australian Journal of International Affairs*, 75, no. 3 (2021): 341–365.

53 Tilak Devasher, 'China's Vaccine One-upmanship', *Tribune*, February 8, 2021, www.tribuneindia.com/news/comment/chinas-vaccine-one-upmanship-209329 (accessed same day); Sanjeev Miglani, 'Vaccine Diplomacy: India Seeks to Rival China with Broad Shipments', Reuters, February 7, 2021 www.reuters.com/a rticle/us-health-coronavirus-india-diplomacy-idUSKBN2A70C8 (accessed on same day); 'COVID-19: Several "Proxy Wars" Spawned by the Pandemic', *News Medical*, April 1, 2021, www.news-medical.net/news/20210401/COVID-19-Several-p roxy-wars-spawned-by-the-pandemic.aspx# (accessed September 29, 2021).

54 Heidi Tworek, 'Competition during Covid-19', in *Competition in World Politics: Knowledge, Strategies and Institutions*, eds Daniela Russ and James Stafford (Verlag, Bielefeld, 2021), 289–299.

55 Ho Benjamin Tze Ern 'Covid-19 and the China Challenge: Interrogating the Domestic-international Nexus in Beijing's Coronavirus Response', *National Security Journal*, 3, no. 3, July 16, 2021 DOI: 10.36878/nsj20210716.01; Marcin Przychodniak, 'The Importance of COVID-19 Vaccines in Chinese Foreign Policy,' *PISM Bulletin*, 48, no. 1744, March 5, 2021, [translated from the original in Polish by Google Translate] https://pism.pl/publications/The_Importance_of_ COVID19_Vaccines_in_Chinese_Foreign_Policy (accessed on October 19, 2021).

56 Ana Nishino, Iori Kawate and Yasuo Takeuchi, 'China Emerges As Big Winner in Vaccine Outreach', Nikkei Asia, April 5, 2021, https://asia.nikkei.com/Sp otlight/Datawatch/China-emerges-as-big-winner-in-vaccine-outreach (accessed on same day); Wu Huizhong and Kristen Gelineau, 'Chinese Vaccines Sweep Much of the World Despite Concerns', AP News, March 2, 2021, https://apnews.com/a rticle/china-vaccines-worldwide-0382aefa52c75b834fbaf6d869808f51 (accessed on September 29, 2021).

57 Peter T.C. Chang, 'China's Vaccine Diplomacy in Malaysia: Problems and Prospects', *Perspective*, September 15, 2021, www.iseas.edu.sg/articles-commentaries/isea s-perspective/2021-121-chinas-vaccine-diplomacy-in-malaysia-problems-and-prospect s-by-peter-t-c-chang/ (accessed on September 29, 2021); Eva Dou and Shibani Mahtani, 'China's Vaccine Diplomacy Stumbles as Clinical Trial Data Remains Absent', *Washington Post*, March 23, 2021, www.washingtonpost.com/world/asia_pacific/ china-coronavirus-singapore-data/2021/03/23/7a0582ca-8afc-11eb-a33e-da28941cb9a c_story.html (accessed on 28 September 2021); Iain Marlow, Archana Choudhary, and Kari Lindberg, 'How India Is Beating China at Its Own Game in Vaccine Diplomacy', NDTV, February 26, 2021, www.ndtv.com/india-news/how-india-is-bea ting-china-at-its-own-game-in-vaccine-diplomacy-2378955 (accessed on same day); James Palmer, 'China's Vaccine Diplomacy Has Mixed Results', *Foreign Policy*, April 7, 2021, https://foreignpolicy.com/2021/04/07/china-coronavirus-vaccine-diploma cy-sinovac-sinopharm-mixed-results/ (accessed on April 8, 2021); Wee Sui-Lee. 'They Relied on Chinese Vaccines. Now They're Battling Outbreaks', *The New York Times*, June 22, 2021, www.nytimes.com/2021/06/22/business/economy/china-vacci

nes-covid-outbreak.html?campaign_id=2&emc=edit_th_20210623&instance_id=33
607&nl=todaysheadlines&regi_id=30381051&segment_id=61450&user_id=fa090c
c506ce13db9a05faea5d295a62 (accessed on same day).

58 'Chinese Vaccines' Effectiveness Low, Official Admits', Al Jazeera, April 12, 2021,
www.aljazeera.com/news/2021/4/11/chinese-vaccines-effectiveness-low-official-admits
(accessed September 30, 2021); 'Covid: WHO Urges China to Co-operate Better in
Virus Origin Probe,' BBC News, July 16, 2021, www.bbc.com/news/world-asia-china
-57855653 (accessed on same day); Dany Shoham, 'The Roots of the COVID-19
Pandemic', BESA Center Perspectives Paper No. 1,847. December 14, 2020, https://
besacenter.org/covid-pandemic-roots/ (accessed on September 30, 2021); Nicholas
Wade, 'The Origin of COVID: Did People or Nature Open Pandora's Box at
Wuhan?', *Bulletin of the Atomic Scientists*, May 5, 2021, https://thebulletin.org/2021/
05/the-origin-of-covid-did-people-or-nature-open-pandoras-box-at-wuhan/ (accessed
May 21, 2021).

59 Christophe Jaffrelot, transl. Cynthis Schoch, *Modi's India: Hindu Nationalism and the
Rise of Ethnic Democracy* (Princeton and Oxford: Princeton University Press, 2021).

60 Mark Tully, 'Securing India's International Image', *Hindustan Times*, February 27,
2021, www.hindustantimes.com/opinion/securing-india-s-international-image-101614
436752809.html (accessed on same day).

4 The Covid-19 Pandemic and Deepening Marginalization in Sri Lanka

Andrea Malji

Introduction

Sri Lanka reported its first Covid-19 case on January 27, 2020, when a Chinese national was admitted to the Infectious Disease Hospital in Angoda.[1] By the second week of March, the first local case was reported in a Sri Lankan tour guide with no history of international travel.[2] Following the first local case, Sri Lanka took swift action to help mitigate the spread of the viral infection. By March 23 the Sri Lankan military had built 45 quarantine centers and used contact-tracing measures to identify and quarantine 14,000 at-risk individuals who came into contact with a Covid-19-positive patient. By March 20, 2020 the state implemented strict measures including an island-wide school closure, work from home measures, a travel ban from selected countries, social distancing measures, and an island wide curfew.[3] The state's initial first-wave response received global recognition by the GRID index, which tracks the Global Leadership Response to Covid-19.[4] Sri Lanka slowly lifted some restrictions beginning in late April and early May only to reintroduce tighter restrictions in late May to help restrict gathering and movement during the Muslim holiday of Eid al-Fitr.[5]

Sri Lanka was able to successfully limit cases during the first wave (March 2020–October 2020), with a weekly average of approximately six cases per day by October 4, 2020 and only 13 deaths during the seven-month period.[6] Sri Lanka entered the second wave of its Covid-19 outbreak beginning in October 2020. Cases and fatalities began to increase, owing to mutations in the virus, particularly the B.1.42 lineage.[7] Despite the rising cases during the second wave, the government did not implement a national lockdown like the one seen during the first wave. Instead, the government utilized targeted responses implementing curfews and short-term district-wide quarantines in the locations with associated clusters (Press Trust of India 2020).[8] With fewer restrictions in place and higher transmissible variants, Sri Lanka's case count and deaths increased dramatically during the second wave. By January 2021 Sri Lanka averaged nearly 4,000 new cases each week, more than it previously experienced in an entire month.[9] The new infection cases decreased somewhat by early April 2021 amid neighboring India's dramatic

DOI: 10.4324/9781003248149-4

spike in Covid-19 cases, owing to the emergence of the highly transmissible Delta variant. However, Sri Lanka's third wave beginning in May 2021 appeared to follow India's dramatic rise in reported cases and deaths. Sri Lanka averaged nearly 13,000 cases per week by the first week of May.[10]

The third wave (May–October 2021) also brought a dramatic increase in Covid-19-related deaths. By May 2021 nearly 50 Sri Lankans a day were dying from Covid-19, and daily fatalities were now higher than the total number of deaths during the first wave. By late July more than 200 Sri Lankans were dying daily.[11] The rapid increase in deaths and pressure from health officials led the reluctant government to reinstate an island-wide lockdown on August 20. The lockdown included the most restrictions the island had seen since the first days of the pandemic. By the time of the new lockdown, Sri Lanka was facing numerous additional crises, both social and economic. Once the August lockdown went into place, Sri Lanka had among the highest Covid-19 death rates in the world.[12] By September the deaths and infection rates remained high, with 483,000 Covid-19 cases since the start of the pandemic and 11,152 deaths. At the height of the third wave, the country of some 21 million was averaging nearly 200 deaths per day. Despite the high rates of positive cases and deaths, the number of cases and deaths might be underreported.[13]

The military and police were central to the initial Covid-19 response, which Sri Lanka scholars have labeled a "statist" approach.[14] The military built and managed quarantine centers while the police enforced curfews and responded to violators. During the initial lockdown period (March–June 2020), Sri Lanka arrested some 56,000 curfew violators and seized 13,556 vehicles that were traveling without a curfew permit.[15] Reports of abuse by police also surged as Covid-19 was used to justify authoritarian responses toward the public. One report claimed that the government selectively used curfew and public health restrictions to target specific communities, such as selective lockdowns of Muslim and low-income communities.[16] Sri Lanka's Inspector General also ordered police to arrest those criticizing the government's coronavirus response.[17]

The strong-armed response by Sri Lanka's security forces is not surprising given the history of militarization, abuse, and human rights violations in the country. Much of the country's post-independence landscape has been defined by exclusionary policies, violence, and nationalism. Those same historical forces seem to be shaping the Covid-19 experience in Sri Lanka.

Sri Lanka's Covid-19 response

The Covid-19 pandemic occurred during a pivotal time in Sri Lanka's political landscape. Sri Lanka found itself at a crossroads following nearly 30 years of civil war that reinforced deep ethnic and religious divisions.[18] Despite a foray into what appeared to be a promising step toward democratic openness, those hopes were quickly dashed by internal political upheaval and the Easter attacks in 2019 carried out by Islamist group National Thowheeth Jama'ath.[19] The attacks occurred amid rising tensions between Sri Lanka's Muslim population and the increasingly influential hardline Buddhist nationalist movement, particularly the Bodu Bala Sena (BBS). Existing tensions between the Sinhalese and Tamil population were further reinforced during this time as well. To understand how these dynamics came to influence Sri Lanka's Covid-19 response, it is necessary to first review how they developed over time.

Background

The Institutionalization of Anti-Minorityism

Sri Lanka has been characterized by deep ethnic, linguistic, and religious divides since before independence. These divisions were shaped by Sri Lanka's colonial history and accelerated during the post-colonial environment. During the colonial era, the British favored Tamils and integrated them into the bureaucracy, educated them in English, and provided extensive training and resources for them. As a result, the Tamils in Sri Lanka became highly represented in the colonial bureaucracy, universities, and armed forces, and were part of Sri Lanka's educated and upwardly mobile class.[20] At the same time, Sri Lanka's Muslim population (often referred to as Moors) were also experiencing economic success, owing to their close involvement in trade and merchantry. The success of the Tamils and the Moors led many Sinhalese Buddhists, who constituted nearly 75% of the population, to question why minority groups within Sri Lanka were experiencing greater levels of success than them. The growing number of Christian conversions at the behest of active Christian missionaries further escalated concerns among the Sinhalese Buddhists about their heritage being erased by outside forces.

Influential 20th-century Sinhalese Buddhist nationalist thinkers such as Anagarika Dharmapala wrote about how the island paradise had been progressively destroyed by outside invaders, from Tamil Nadu, the Arab world, and then the West.[21] Dharmapala argued that collectively these groups contributed to the cultural decline of Sinhalese Buddhism and would soon dominate control while the original inhabitants of the island languished. His rhetoric helped inspire and mobilize Buddhist nationalists who wanted to reclaim Sri Lanka for Sinhalese Buddhists. Although the Sinhalese and Tamils had tensions during the colonial era, their leaders were relatively united to defeat the colonial occupation and had focused on both Sinhala and Tamil as national languages to replace English.[22]

Once the country gained independence in 1948, the power dynamics quickly transitioned to diminish Tamil power and increase Sinhalese superimposition. Political Buddhism became increasingly prevalent in national politics. Buddhist monks (*Bhikkus*) considered involvement in Sri Lankan politics to be a social duty and reflective of the historical ties between the monks and Kings.[23] The language of the *Bhikkus* was divisive and helped nurture support for Sinhalization policies over the following years beginning with the transformational 1956 election whereby S.W.R.D. Bandaranaike and the Sri Lanka Freedom Party (SLFP) campaigned on a Sinhala only platform.[24] The SLFP had developed an increasingly close relationship with the Buddhist monks who sought to institutionalize Buddhist ethics and practices and fuse language (Sinhala) and religion.[25] The same year that the SLFP won a convincing election, they instituted the Sinhala Only Act, which replaced English as the official language, which was not spoken by approximately 29% of the country at the time. Over the following years under the SLFP, several anti-Tamil, pro-Sinhalese nationalist acts were passed including quotas in universities and jobs for Sinhalese, settlement of Sinhalese in Tamil areas, and giving Buddhism the "foremost place" in the 1972 constitution.[26] Additional incidents of anti-Tamil violence and pogroms throughout the country gave rise to the counter-nationalist movement by the Tamils which would escalate into an eventual civil war between the Liberation Tamil Tigers Eelam (LTTE) and the Sri Lanka government following the Black July pogrom in 1983.[27]

The Civil War lasted from 1983 until 2009 and killed approximately 100,000 people and led to the disappearance of tens of thousands more.[28] Nearly one million Tamils also fled the island during this time.[29] During the civil war, Buddhist nationalist policies and rhetoric became increasingly prevalent and public Buddhist iconography became more common and associated with the Sri Lankan war effort.[30] At the same time, many monks promoted the use of strong military force against the LTTE, some monks even ran for office through the Jathika Hela Urumaya (JHU) party to promote their militant platforms.[31] The JHU failed to gain much momentum, and the nationalist monks instead found comfort coalescing with the Rajapaksa family, with Mahinda Rajapaksa as President and his brother Gotabaya as Minister of Defense from 2005 until 2015.[32] The Rajapaksa brothers weaponized the support from the Buddhist nationalists throughout the country to implement their brutal response to the final phase of the civil war, which resulted in widespread killing of civilians, and what human rights organizations have labeled war crimes and widespread human rights violations.[33]

Despite what many Buddhist nationalists might consider to be a decisive victory, following the end of the civil war Buddhist nationalist forces became increasingly mobilized and politically active.[34] However, the nature of the mobilization by Buddhist forces took a distinctive turn to now focus on the minority Muslim community.[35] Although early Buddhist nationalist discourse espoused by those such as Dharmapala included a particular anti-Muslim angle, Muslims had mostly been excluded from the fractionalization that defined the Sinhalese and Tamil communities. In fact, most Muslims had generally supported the state efforts during the civil war.[36] As the war ended, organizations like the BBS sought to emulate the same type of religious nationalistic community mobilization seen in other countries like the 969 movement and Ma Ba Tha movement in Myanmar and the Rashtriya Swayamsevak Sangh in India (Holt 2016). Buddhist monks and BBS leaders began holding rallies decrying the risk Muslims pose to Sri Lanka. BBS' leader Galagoda-Atte Gnanasara Thero began holding increasingly divisive rallies using anti-Muslim rhetoric and slurs:

> "In this country we still have a Sinhala police; we still have a Sinhala army. After today if a single Marakkalaya (slur for Muslims) or some other paraya (alien) touches a single Sinhalese….it will be their end."[37]

The speech, which occurred in Aluthgama following an altercation between Muslim youths and a Sinhalese lorry driver that left the driver dead, featured a call to action converting the crowd into a mob. Within hours of Thero's address, anti-Muslim riots broke out throughout the region destroying Muslim businesses and damaging mosques, four were killed, eighty were injured, and more than 10,000 displaced.[38] The UNHCR released a statement following the attacks, saying it is alarmed by the intercommunal violence and hate speech.[39]

The 2015 election of Maithripala Sirisena, which ousted Rajapaksa, momentarily assuaged concerns about the rising anti-Muslim environment throughout Sri Lanka. Brief liberalization policies and attempts at reconciliation with the Tamil community promised to transform the divided Sri Lanka. However, this reprieve was short lived as anti-Muslim mobs carried out attacks in February and March 2018 throughout Ampara and Kandy. Security forces did little to stop the anti-Muslim riots, and some even participated.[40] The attacks eventually led the government to declare a state of emergency and social media blackout.[41] The riots occurred following false social media rumors saying that Muslim business owners were covertly sterilizing the Sinhalese population. The 2018 riots were a watershed moment that allegedly inspired the formation of the National Thowheeth Jama'ath, who went on to carry out one of Sri Lanka's deadliest attacks in Easter 2019, killing 269 and injuring more than 500.[42]

The Easter attacks were a breaking point in the future of Sri Lanka's political destiny. Buddhist nationalists called for harsh reprisals and anti-terrorism measures by the government. The attacks created an opening for the return of the Rajapaksa brothers offering to re-enter the political scene and run for office. Gotabaya Rajapaksa's historical hawkishness appealed to Buddhist nationalists throughout the country that wanted to utilize his historical military brutality to defeat the growing Islamic terrorism problem within the country. Radical Buddhist monks, including the BBS, strongly supported the Rajapaksa 2019 campaign and utilized exclusionary anti-minority language to promote Rajapaksa's candidacy.[43] Not surprisingly Rajapaksa easily won the election. Gotabaya's brother and former president Mahinda Rajapaksa was appointed Prime Minister shortly after the Covid-19 pandemic arrived in Sri Lanka just two months after Rajapaksa's win. Not surprisingly, the Rajapaksa government took several authoritarian positions amid the outbreak to discriminate against minorities and institutionalize anti-minority programs targeting both Tamils and Muslims.

Covid-19 and the Consolidation of Exclusionary Policies

The Covid-19 outbreak arrived upon the heels of increasing communal tensions between the Sinhalese and Muslim community. Likewise, despite a decrease in Tamil-Sinhalese tensions following the 2009 cessation of the Civil War, pervasive anti-Tamil policies, including restriction on movement, forced disappearances, and torture, also re-emerged. A cross section of literature has demonstrated that regimes might utilize emergencies to consolidate authoritarian policies.[44] The Easter attacks and the Covid-19 crisis have allowed the Rajapaksa regime to consolidate their discriminatory policies in the name of both public health and safety and security. The division has been so notable that a 2021 UN report on the human rights situation within the country noted that despite initial success in containing the Covid-19 pandemic, the social and economic impact has been "deep and exacerbated social disparities."[45]

The 2015 presidential election of Rajapaksa cabinet defector Maithripala Sirisena appeared to be a key turning point in Sri Lanka's domestic affairs. Sirisena came to power on a reconciliatory platform including a promise to investigate war crimes carried out during the final phases of the civil war.[46] During Sirisena's tenure, the Sri Lankan government made historic progress by cosponsoring and complying with the UN Human Rights Council Resolution 30/1, which committed Sri Lanka to reconciliation efforts by establishing independent judiciary committees to investigate allegations of human rights abuse.[47] During the same year the government also made important steps toward reconciliation by including the Tamil national anthem in Independence Day events, which had not happened since the early years of independence.[48] The brief optimism that came along with Sirisena's election quickly unraveled during the country's 2018 constitutional crisis.[49] Sirisena dismissed Prime Minister Wickremesinghe and installed Mahinda Rajapaksa—a move that opposition parties protested as unconstitutional. Sirisena attempted to suspend Parliament and convince the PM's party to support Rajapaksa as the new Prime Minister. Sirisena was unable to succeed and Wickremesinghe retained his position, owing to the support of his United National Party and the Tamil and Muslim minority parties. Although unsuccessful, the event demonstrated the democratic backsliding under the Sirisena regime, which Freedom House coined a failed coup attempt.[50]

Sri Lanka's deadly easter terrorist attacks by Islamic extremist group National Thowheeth Jama'ath six months later in effect halted reconciliation efforts. In response, the government quickly utilized the civil war-era Prevention of Terrorism Act to detain Muslim suspects throughout the country. Although the November 2019 election of Gotabaya Rajapaksa marked the escalation of anti-minority policies, the arrival of Covid-19 allowed the regime to justify its authoritarian policies amid the concurrent threats of terrorism and pandemic. Consequently, policies and protocols done in the name of public safety have been used to enact anti-minority measures, restrict movement, and delay elections.

Prior to Sri Lanka's island-wide shutdown and curfew, President Rajapaksa created a task force to create a "disciplined, virtuous, and lawful society. "[51] As part of this task force, Rajapaksa increasingly militarized civilian institutions and appointed family members into key roles, including disaster management.[52] Since then, increased police abuse has been reported throughout the island. Multiple curfew and quarantine breakers have been arrested, tortured, and/or killed. Human Rights Watch noted that police began increasingly using Covid-19 measures as justification to kill and abuse citizens.[53] The Covid-19 restrictions were also used to detain peaceful protestors, which led the Bar Association of Sri Lanka to condemn the police's use of the pandemic to "curtail freedom of expression."[54]

Once parliamentary elections were held, Rajapaksa's party won in a landslide. However, elections were delayed for several months. Just days before the World Health Organization (WHO) declared a global pandemic, President Rajapaksa dissolved Parliament six months early and called for early elections on April 25 2020.[55] Despite Sri Lanka's low Covid-19 numbers in April 2020, the National Election Committee delayed the April 25 elections until June 20 and then again until August 5, in the name of public health.[56] Following the election delays, Mahinda Rajapaksa's party won a super-majority and was sworn into office by his brother Gotabaya at a Buddhist temple in Colombo.[57] Following the victory, Rajapaksa passed the 20th amendment, which expanded the powers of the Presidency.[58]

National elections were not the only delayed democratic events. In December 2020, the government postponed Provincial Council elections, owing to the rising Covid-19 cases. Provincial councils were established during the Indo-Lanka Peace Accords in 1987 to help devolve power to the provincial level as part of a reconciliation effort put forth by Sri Lanka's 13th amendment.[59] Unlike the national elections that were eventually held after delays, provincial elections have been repeatedly delayed with no new election date announced, although government leaders said it will happen by the end of 2021.[60] The delay in the provincial elections with no commitment to a new date comes amid comments from Sri Lanka's High Commissioner-designate to India, who called the provincial councils "superfluous, expensive, divisive," and said that it is "fraught with inefficiency."[61] These comments indicate that the pandemic might be used as an excuse to minimize or indefinitely delay reconciliation efforts, particularly provincial councils, which are highly opposed by right wing nationalist forces in Sri Lanka.

While the pandemic has led Sri Lanka to introduce and escalate authoritarian measures broadly, it has specifically been utilized to target the two main minority groups within the country, Muslims and Tamils. Essentially, Covid-19 has been weaponized to institutionalize discriminatory policies and human rights violations.

Targeting of Muslims

Sri Lanka's anti-democratic provisions during the pandemic have been rife with communal undertones. Not only has the government used the pandemic to limit specific post-civil war reconciliation commitments, such as the provincial councils, it has also enacted anti-minority policies that organizations such as the Muslim Council of Sri Lanka have called racist.[62] One specific discriminatory policy enacted in April 2020 was Sri Lanka's policy of compulsory cremation of Covid-19 victims.[63] In Islam, cremation is considered a forbidden practice that desecrates the body.[64] The forced cremation policy was a reversal in Sri Lanka's earlier health guidelines from the Sri Lankan Ministry of Health, which stated that those who died from Covid-19 should not be washed or touched but placed in a sealed bag in a coffin The earlier guidelines also stated that in addition to cremation, burial was allowed, as long as ground water was not impacted.[65] Cremation is the preferred practice of Hindus and Buddhists, which constitute nearly 90% of the island. However, since the early days of the pandemic, the WHO among other organizations have made it clear that cremation is not required drawing attention to their earlier guidelines that "there are no health advantages of cremation over burial."[66] The UN High Commissioner on Human Rights said Sri Lanka's policy "failed to respect the religious feelings of the victims and their family members, especially Muslims, Catholics, and some Buddhists."[67]

The policy of forced cremation continued for nearly a year and was apparently abetted following an official state visit by Pakistan's Prime Minister Imran Khan in February 2021. Khan noted his opposition to the policy and Sri Lanka abandoned it shortly after.[68] This concession came as Sri Lanka sought international support against the upcoming March 2021 United Nations vote regarding investigation into Sri Lanka's alleged war crimes. Pakistan subsequently voted against the request to enhance monitoring of the human rights situation in Sri Lanka.[69] Despite abandoning the cremation policy, the country still utilized exclusionary measures for families choosing to bury their Covid-19 victims. Initially, victims' families were required to use a government designated burial site on Iranathivu island, an isolated area in the Tamil dominated north. Tamil families also protested the decision which led the government to eventually remove the area as a burial site option in favor of a burial ground in Muslim majority Batticaloa, in eastern Sri Lanka.[70] Buddhist nationalists continued to call for mandatory cremation, saying that burials of Covid-19 victims would corrupt the sacred land and risked being weaponized.[71]

The anti-Muslim policies came amid a rise in broader government persecution of the Muslim community since the Easter 2019 attacks. Shortly after the island wide curfew was implemented in early April 2020, authorities arrested a prominent Muslim lawyer that had challenged the government's anti-Muslim policies, particularly during the pandemic.[72] Six other high-ranking Muslim community members were also arrested in a government sweep.[73] One of the arrested, Ramzy Razeek, was a retired government official who publicly characterized the government's Covid-19 cremation policy as religious discrimination. Ramzeek was held for allegedly "advocating hatred leading to incitement to hostility, discrimination, or violence."[74] Once detained, medical treatment and regular access to lawyers were denied, allegedly owing to concerns about Covid-19.

The early cases in Muslim majority area were heavily emphasized and overrepresented in media reports on the virus in Sri Lanka.[75] Sri Lankan Muslims noted an even further uptick in hate speech, boycotts, surveillance, and rumors, once the pandemic started.[76] This was aided by speeches from government and military leaders that attempted to tie Muslims to Covid-19 spread by stating that a majority of Covid-19 patients on island were Muslim. Sri Lanka's Minister of Health even stated that the island would have been able to celebrate Avurudu (Sinhalese New Year) if not for the remaining Covid-19 cases, who were Muslim.[77] The accusations held similarities to the widespread critique of Muslims, specifically the Tablighi Jamaat in India, who were blamed for the spread of Covid-19 in India.[78] Following these public statements, Muslim events were seen as "super spreader events."[79] Sinhalese Buddhists were warned not to buy food items from Muslim vendors. Shutdowns and surveillance specifically targeting Muslim towns such as Etulgama, Beruwala, and Akurana were also reported.[80]

The pandemic also allowed the government to reinstate previous policies that singled out the Muslim population. One example is the April 2021 reinstatement of the face-veil and niqab ban. The Minister of Public Security Sarath Weerasekera claimed that face veils and the *burqa*, are a sign of religious extremism and a threat to national security.[81] The government had temporarily banned face veils in 2019 following the Easter attacks, claiming it a necessary step amid an urgent national security crisis. Muslim officials and human rights activists from around the world criticized the ban.[82] The UN special rapporteur on freedom of said the ban is a violation of international law and religious freedom of expression.[83] Despite the public health crisis, the government used the pandemic to implement controversial exclusionary policies, strategically this reduced public criticism because criticism of the government during a national crisis could result in a number of negative responses by the state, including detention.

Anti-Muslim rhetoric and actions toward Sri Lankan Muslims during the Covid-19 pandemic were an extension of an ongoing and escalating problem in the country. The pandemic allowed the government to institutionalize exclusionary policies in the name of public safety. Misinformation via social media toward the Muslim community helped to further escalate anti-Muslim bias. However, Sri Lankan Muslims have not been alone in the targeting. The Tamil community also continued to face persecution from the government during the pandemic, including the all too familiar tactics of torture, kidnapping, and restriction of movement.

Targeting of Tamils

Many refer to the period following the end of the Sri Lankan civil war as the post-conflict era. When I used this term during fieldwork in 2019, I was quickly corrected by Tamil residents. One respondent reminded me that the end of the war doesn't mean the end of the conflict. A human rights activist told me that Tamils still face high levels of persecution, they are just murdered less frequently than before. International observers tend to agree with this assessment, a 2021 report on human rights in Sri Lanka, the UN called attention to Sri Lanka's "progressively deepening discrimination and marginalization of the country's minorities."[84]

When the war ended an estimated 100,000 Tamils had died in the conflict and nearly one million fled the country.[85] The war decimated much of the land and population, making reconstruction difficult. Reconciliation efforts seemed bleak following the brutality that ended the war. However, as previously mentioned, some hope appeared with the election of Sirisena in 2015. Specifically, Sri Lanka's 2015 co-sponsorship of UNHCR resolution 30/1 gave some temporary relief to Tamils. In addition, the 2015 death sentence of Army Staff Sergeant Sunil Rathnayake for his role in a massacre of Tamils in 2000 indicated the government's willingness to prosecute war crimes.[86] Sirisena also halted Sinhalese resettlement schemes that provided land, housing, and infrastructure for Sinhalese that relocated to Tamil majority areas.[87] On an important cultural note, the Tamil national anthem was included in 2016 Independence Day events for the first time since 1949.[88] This inclusion offered additional evidence of easing tensions and inclusion.

This progress began backsliding even before Sirisena's term ended, but the November 2019 Presidential election of Rajapaksa eliminated many progressive steps. With Covid-19 reaching the country within two months of his election, Rajapaksa was able to utilize the pandemic to implement draconian measures. Additionally, with the primary local and global focus on the pandemic, there was less scrutiny for divisive measures taken by the regime. Rajapaksa's militarization of the civilian sector further ensured there was minimal internal and external criticism of his policies.

One of the first measures indicating Rajapaksa's lack of commitment to reconciliation was Sri Lanka's February 2020 withdrawal from the UN Human Rights Council's justice and reconciliation process. Next, the removal of the Tamil national anthem from Independence Day events in February 2020 indicated a key cultural shift. The removal of the Tamil national anthem was even noted by the UN High Commissioner of Human Rights, who noted in her report to the UN on Sri Lanka's human rights conditions that:

"The Government declined to include the National Anthem in the Tamil language on national occasions, such as the Independence Day celebrations, on 4 February 2020, despite the preceding years' practice of singing it in two languages as a significant gesture towards reconciliation."[89]

Sri Lanka's Minister of Defense responded to the report saying that it was "very pathetic," "full of nonsense", and based on "bogus information."[90] At the same Independence Day events Rajapaksa alluded to his commitment to unity, saying "as the president today, I represent the entire Sri Lankan nation irrespective of ethnicity, religion, party affiliation or other differences."[91] However, in practice, there still appears to be two different realities based on one's ethnicity and religion. For example, while campaigning for President, Gotabaya Rajapaksa claimed that once in power he would acquit "war heroes" that were held on "baseless charges."[92] Then, in March 2020, just days into the island-wide lockdown, Rajapaksa gave a presidential pardon to Sunil Ratyanake, who had been sentenced to death in 2015, owing to his torture and murder of eight Tamil civilians.[93] Ratyanake's appeals for release were denied by the Supreme Court as recently as 2019.[94] However, Rajapaksa overrode the court's ruling and carried out the pardon amid the height of public paranoia surrounding Covid-19.

The resettlement of Sinhalese families into Tamil majority areas has also escalated during the pandemic. The United Nations Human Rights Commission has stated that resettlement of internally displaced persons from the war is a key component of reconciliation in the country. However, instead of resettlement of Tamils, the government has utilized "irrigation schemes, military settlements, archaeological reservations, wildlife sanctuaries, forest reserves and special economic zones" to accelerate land-grabbing in the North and East.[95] Despite restrictions on movements during the lockdown, dozens of Sinhalese farmers have relocated to historically Tamil areas alongside several new Buddhist temples.[96] However, for Tamils in the north and east, once Covid-19 hit, restrictions on movement became increasingly difficult. The traditional livelihood of many Tamil fishermen was restricted, owing to the curfew, with limited aid being distributed by the government to the fishing communities. Military checkpoints also increased, particularly in Tamil and Muslim areas and prevented movement of Tamil civilians, despite a lack of access to basic goods such as clean water.[97] The increased militarization and lack of access into the region for human rights organizations and non-governmental organizations limited their ability to observe possible violations.

In addition to widespread curfew restrictions and limitations on movement, Tamils reported the ongoing destruction and threat of destruction of archaeological sites. The destruction of heritage sites has long been used as a strategy of nationalism to help reclaim disputed space for the dominant ethno-religious group.[98] The attempt to reclaim Buddhist sites from Hindus and Muslims had already been escalating before the pandemic.[99] Then, in June 2020, Rajapaksa appointed an all-Sinhala archaeological council that sought to identify and reclaim Buddhist heritage sites in Tamil and Muslim dominated areas. Nearly half the council members are Buddhist monks with no archaeological expertise and none of the council members are Tamil or Muslims.[100] The council continued to operate during the pandemic and identify heritage sites that might contain historical Buddhist artifacts. By 2021 the task force identified and reclaimed items from dozens of sites just in Muslim dominated Batticaloa district that allegedly contained Buddhist historical items.[101] In addition to forming a task force to investigate sites, the government has also actively destroyed sites and memorials. In January 2021 the government destroyed a Tamil war memorial at Jaffna university, further weakening attempts at reconciliation.[102] The government eventually agreed to rebuild it following strong backlash including hunger strikes by students and activists.[103] However, these actions are taking place while there is limited international observers, threats of arrest for criticizing the government Covid-19 response, restrictions on movement, and active Sinhalese resettlement campaigns. Minorities in Sri Lanka already have limited power, but the pandemic has been utilized to limit dissent, arrest critics, minimize assemblies and protests, limit freedom of movement, enact stricter surveillance, and further weaponize archaeology. These tactics are all part of a broader attempt to further Sinhalize minority areas.

The twin threats of the pandemic and terrorism have allowed the government to further implement authoritarian measures in the name of safety and security. The UNHCR reported that the pandemic has been used to "justify excessive or arbitrary limits on legitimate freedom of expression and association." For example, the pandemic was cited as justification for the ban on visitation by legal representatives. Those arrested under the Terrorism Prevention Act were supposedly left in poor conditions without access to healthcare or their legal representatives.[104]

Even when restrictions loosened and larger gatherings were allowed, government critics and minorities were punitively targeted. In February 2021, thousands of activists, politicians, and students took the streets to participate in the Pothuvil to Polikandy (P2P) march for justice. The rally marched through cities impacted by the war and what the activists called "Sinhalization" policies. The rally took place following months of restricted movement owing to the pandemic and sought to draw attention to various violations by the government including increased Sinhalese settlements in Tamil areas, forced disappearances of activists, increasing militarization during the pandemic, intimidation of activists and journalists, the misuse of the Prevention of Terrorism Act to target ethnic and religious minorities, and the detention of political prisoners without trial.[105] Several participants were arrested for their participation in the march. In September 2021, a report from the International Truth and Justice Project found that detainees from the P2P march and other vigil events were beaten, burnt, and sexually abused by the authorities.[106] The report notes that torture and disappearances continue even during Covid-19, and once arrested the detainees have limited rights to visitation or court proceedings, owing to the pandemic. Despite limitations on visitors, the government has been unable to control the spread of Covid-19 in prisons, with high numbers of detainees testing positive, which even escalated into a Covid-19 related riot within one prison that left eight prisoners dead and dozens injured (Reuters 2020). In September 2021 one government minister even entered the prison to abuse Tamil inmates, forcing them to kneel at gunpoint and then assaulting them.[107]

Conditions within prison facilities and throughout minority dominated areas of Sri Lanka remain poor and reflect an ongoing degradation of human rights within the country. The situation has not only worsened for minorities, but the spectrum of who is targeted has also broadened. As the UN Human Rights Commissioner has recently affirmed, during the Covid-19 pandemic, "surveillance, intimidation and judicial harassment of human rights defenders, journalists and families of the disappeared has not only continued but has broadened to a wider spectrum of students, academics, medical professionals and religious leaders critical of government policies."[108]

Conclusion: Increasing Militarization Spurred by the Pandemic

The Covid-19 response in Sri Lanka has predominantly been administered by the military and police. The security forces have been given a tremendous responsibility that limits civilian oversight of their pandemic protocols. Because of this, reports of police abuses have surged, with specific targeting of ethnic and religious minorities. Police have been linked to several deaths in custody of Covid-19 quarantine violators in addition to reports of abusive enforcement.[109] The deaths and abuses of Sri Lankans, particularly in Tamil and Muslim areas have led human right groups, the UN, and the Bar Association of Sri Lanka to condemn the use of police force and retaliation toward detainees and peaceful protestors, including those outside quarantine facilities.

Despite initial successes in stopping the spread, Sri Lanka is facing several emergencies nearly two years into the pandemic. By September 2021 Sri Lanka had recorded a drastic increase in cases and deaths, with some 417,000 cases and nearly12,680 deaths, with among the highest case fatality ratios in the world as of September 2021.[110] To worsen the situation, the country declared a food emergency on August 30, 2021, owing to the lack of foreign exchange funding to finance imports.[111] The new emergency regulations, enforced by a military general, allow the government to seize food stocks and arrest from those deemed to be hoarding supplies.

Sri Lanka has been characterized by increasing militarization since the November 2019 election of Rajapaksa. The pandemic has allowed the government to increase and institutionalize exclusionary policies, often in the name of protecting public health. Some of the initial reconciliatory successes of post-conflict Sri Lanka have quickly dissipated. In exchange, the Easter 2019 attacks and Covid-19 have combined to reinforce and even amplify old ethnic and religious divides. Sri Lanka's history of ethnic conflict serves as a warning about how these fractionalizations can escalate. If the government continues to avoid reconciliation efforts these disputes will only deepen and threaten to destabilize the country.

Notes

1   Reuters, 'Sri Lanka Confirms First Case of Coronavirus', January 27, 2020.
2   Press Trust of India, '52-year-old tour guide from Sri Lanka is the country's first coronavirus patient', *First Post*, March 11, 2020.
3   Dilanthi Amaratunga et al, 'The COVID-19 Outbreak in Sri Lanka: A Synoptic Analysis Focusing on Trends, Impacts, Risks and Science-Policy Interaction Processes', *Progress in Disaster Science* (2020).
4   Ibid.
5   'Sri Lanka Lifts Nationwide Lockdown.' *The Hindu*, June 28, 2020.
6   Ensheng Dong, Hongru Du, and Lauren Gardner. 'An Interactive Web-Based Dashboard to Track COVID 19 in Real Time.' *The Lancet Infectious Diseases*, 20, no. 5 (2020): 533–534.
7   World Health Organization. 'Environmental Health in Emergencies: Technical Notes on Water and Sanitation.' March 2007.
8   Press Trust of India, 'Sri Lanka's second COVID-19 wave has high transmissibility: Study', *New Indian Express*, October 31, 2020.
9   Dong, Du, and Gardner, 'An Interactive Web-Based Dashboard.'
10 Ibid.
11 Ibid.
12 Ibid.
13 Soban Qadir Khan et al. 'Under-reported COVID-19 cases in South Asian Countries.' *F1000Research*, 10 (2021).
14 Kalinga Silva, 'Identity, Infection, and Fear: A Preliminary Analysis of COVID-19 Drivers and Responses in Sri Lanka,' International Center for Ethnic Studies (2020).
15 News First, 'More than 13,000 Curfew Violators Arrested as Sri Lanka Enters Nationwide Curfew', May 17, 2020.
16 Silva, 'Identity, Infection, and Fear'.
17 Meenakshi Ganguly, 'Sri Lanka Uses Pandemic to Curtail Free Expression', Human Rights Watch, April 3,2020.
18 Rachel Seoighe, *War, Denial and Nation-Building in Sri Lanka: After the End*, Springer (2017).
19 Amarnath Amarasingham, 'Terrorism on the Teardrop Island: Understanding the Easter 2019 Attacks in Sri Lanka', *CTC Sentinel*, 12, no. 5 (2019): 1–10.
20 Neil DeVotta, 'Sinhalese Buddhist Nationalist Ideology: Implications for Politics and Conflict Resolution in Sri Lanka.' East West Center, Policy Studies, No. 40 (2007).
21 Mikael Gravers, 'Anti-Muslim Buddhist Nationalism in Burma and Sri Lanka: Religious Violence and Globalized Imaginaries of Endangered Identities,' *Contemporary Buddhism*, 16, no. 1 (2015): 1–27.
22 Neil DeVotta, Blowback: Linguistic Nationalism, Institutional Decay, and Ethnic Conflict in Sri Lanka (Stanford: Stanford University Press, 2004).
23 Walpola Rahula, History of Buddhism in Ceylon-The Anuradhapura Period, 3rd century BC-10th century AD (Colombo, M.D. Gunasena & Co., 1956).
24 Neil DeVotta, 'The Genesis, Consolidation, and Consequences of Sinhalese Buddhist Nationalism,' in *When Politics Are Sacralized: Comparative Perspectives on Religious Claims and Nationalism* (2021): 187.
25 Ibid.
26 DeVotta, *Blowback*.
27 Michael Roberts, *Exploring Confrontation: Sri Lanka: Politics, Culture and History* (Oxfordshire: Routledge, 2021).
28 BBC. 'Sri Lanka Civil War: Rajapaksa says Thousands Missing are Dead.' January 20, 2020.

29 Arun Kumar Acharya, 'Ethnic Conflict and Refugees in Sri Lanka.' *Antropología Experimental*, 7 (2007).

30 Chamindra Weerawardhana, 'Paradigms of [In] Tolerance? On Sri Lanka's Bodu Bala Sena, #prezpollsl2015, and Transformative Dynamics of Lived Religion.' In *Lived Religion and the Politics of (In) Tolerance* (London: Palgrave Macmillan, 2017), 19–39.

31 Neil DeVotta, and Jason Stone. 'Jathika Heia Urumaya and Ethno-Religious Politics in Sri Lanka.' *Pacific Affairs* (2008): 31–51.

32 John Holt, ed. *Buddhist Extremists and Muslim Minorities: Religious Conflict in Contemporary Sri Lanka* (Oxford: Oxford University Press, 2016).

33 Jayadeva Uyangoda, 'Sri Lanka in 2009: From Civil War to Political Uncertainties', *Asian Survey*, 50, no. 1 (2010): 104–111.

34 DeVotta, 'Sinhalese Buddhist Nationalist Ideologies'.

35 Mikael Gravers, 'Anti-Muslim Buddhist Nationalism in Burma and Sri Lanka: Religious Violence and Globalized Imaginaries of Endangered Identities,' *Contemporary Buddhism*, 16, no. 1 (2015): 1–27.

36 Athambawa Sarjoon, Mohammad Agus Yusoff, and Nordin Hussin, 'Anti-Muslim Sentiments and Violence: A Major Threat to Ethnic Reconciliation and Ethnic Harmony in Post-War Sri Lanka,' *Religions*, 7, no. 10 (2016): 125.

37 Galagoda Aththe Gnanasara Thero (speech, Kandy, Sri Lanka, June 15, 2014)

38 Dilrukshi Handunneti, 'Sri Lanka Muslims Remember Buddhist Hardliner Attacks', Al Jazeera, June 15, 2016.

39 UN News Service, Sri Lanka, 'UN Rights Chief Alarmed at Inter-Communal Violence, Urges End to Hate Speech', June 16, 2014.

40 Tom Allard and Shihar Aneez, 'Police, Politicians Accused of Joining Sri Lanka's anti-Muslim Riots.' Reuters, March 24, 2018.

41 Meenakshi Ganguly, 'State of Emergency Declared in Sri Lanka,' Human Rights Watch, March 7, 2018.

42 Amarnath Amarasingham, 'Terrorism on the Teardrop Island: Understanding the Easter 2019 attacks in Sri Lanka.' *CTC Sentinel*, 12, no. 5 (2019): 1–10

43 Pasan Jayasinghe, 'Hegemonic Populism: Sinhalese Buddhist Nationalist Populism in Contemporary Sri Lanka.' In *Populism in Asian Democracies*, pp. 176–196 (2020).

44 Victor Ramraj, *No Doctrine More Pernicious? Emergencies and the Limits of Legality*, in 'Emergencies and the Limits of Legality', ed. Victor Ramraj, (Cambridge: Cambridge University Press 2008); Austin Sarat, *Toward New Conceptions of the Relationship of Law and Sovereignty under the Conditions of Emergency* in 'Sovereignty, Emergency, Legality', ed. Austin Serat, (Cambridge: Cambridge University Press 2010); Stephen Thomson and Eric C. Ip, 'COVID-19 Emergency Measures and the Impending Authoritarian Pandemic.' *Journal of Law and the Biosciences*, 7, no. 1 (2020).

45 Office of the High Commissioner of Human Rights, 'Sri Lanka on Alarming Path Towards Recurrence of Grave Human Rights Violations-UN Report', January 27, 2021.

46 Jeffrey Feltman, *Sri Lanka's Presidential Elections: Progress, Regression, Or Paralysis?* Brookings Institution (2019).

47 Menik Wakkumbura, 'Challenges to Peacebuilding Approaches: Analysing Sri Lanka's Peace Efforts During the First 10 Years Ending the Civil War', *Journal of Peacebuilding & Development* (2021).

48 Azzam Ameen, 'Sri Lankan Anthem Sung in Tamil for First Time Since 1949', BBC News, February 4, 2016.

49 Andreas Johansson, 'The 2018 Political Crisis and Muslim Politics in Sri Lanka', *ISAS Insight*, 2018.

50 Freedom House, 'Sri Lanka's Democracy Hangs in the Balance after 'Coup Attempt', Freedom House, 2018.

51 DeVotta, 'Sinhalese Buddhist Nationalist Ideologies'.
52 Nira Wickramasinghe, 'Sri Lanka in 2020: Return to Rajapaksa Regnum,' *Asian Survey*, 61, no. 1 (2021): 211–16.
53 Ganguly, 'Sri Lanka Uses Pandemic to Curtail Free Expression.'
54 Bar Association of Sri Lanka, 'Statement by the Executive Committee of the Bar Association of Sri Lanka,' June 10, 2021.
55 Wickramasinghe, 'Sri Lanka in 2020'.
56 Waruna Karunatilake, 'Sri Lanka Delays General Election for Second Time, sets August 5 as New Date.' Reuters, June 10, 2020.
57 Al Jazeera, 'Mahinda Rajapaksa sworn in as Sri Lanka's PM after record victory', August 9, 2020.
58 Wickramasinghe, 'Sri Lanka in 2020'.
59 DeVotta, 'The Genesis, Consolidation, and Consequences'.
60 Arjuna Ranawana, 'PC polls postponement partly due to Right-Wing pressure.' *Economy Next*, December 30, 2020.
61 Tamil Guardian, 'Who Cares, I Served My Country,'– Sri Lanka's Defence Secretary lashes out at UNHRC', February 26, 2021.
62 BBC, 'Covid-19: Sri Lanka Chooses Remote Island for Burials,' March 2, 2021.
63 Althaf Marsoof, 'The Disposal of COVID-19 Dead Bodies: The Impact of Sri Lanka's Response on Fundamental Rights,' *Journal of Human Rights Practice* (2021).
64 Andrea Malji and Amarnath Amarasingham. 'Forced Cremation of Covid Dead in Sri Lanka Further Marginalizes Muslim Community.' *Religion Dispatches*, December 15, 2020.
65 Ibid.
66 World Health Organization, 'Environmental Health in Emergencies: Technical Notes on Water and Sanitation', March (2007).
67 Office of the High Commissioner of Human Rights. 'Sri Lanka: Compulsory Cremation of COVID-19 Bodies Cannot Continue, say UN experts,' January 25, 2021.
68 Press Trust of India. "Sri Lanka Ends Forced Cremations of Covid-19 Victims After Imran Khan's Visit." Hindustan Times, February 26, 2021.
69 UNHRC. '46th session of the Human Rights Council: Resolutions, decisions and President's statements. 46/1 Promoting reconciliation, accountability and human rights in Sri Lanka', March 23, 2021.
70 Colombo Page. 'Government Scraps Idea of Burying Covid Dead in Iranativu Island.' March 8, 2021.
71 BBC, 'Covid-19: Sri Lanka Chooses Remote Island for Burials', March 2, 2021.
72 Human Rights Watch, 'Sri Lanka: Due Process Concerns in Arrests of Muslims,' April 23, 2020.
73 Ibid.
74 Ibid.
75 Silva, 'Identity, Infection, and Fear.'
76 Tisaranee Gunasekara, 'The President in the Pandemic', *Groundviews*, May 5, 2020.
77 Ayesha Zuhair, 'Disinformation is Damaging Sri Lanka's COVID-19 Response', *Daily FT*, April 13, 2020.
78 Roshni Kapur, 'Covid-19 in India and Sri Lanka: New Forms of Islamophobia', Middle East Institute, July 7, 2020.
79 Silva, 'Identity, Infection, and Fear.'
80 Ibid.
81 Al Jazeera, 'Sri Lanka Cabinet Approves Proposed Ban on Burqas in Public', April 28, 2021.
82 Ibid.
83 International Commission of Jurists, 'Sri Lanka: Parliament Must Reject Proposed 'Burqa Ban', April 30, 2021.

84   Office of the High Commissioner of Human Rights, 'Sri Lanka on Alarming Path Towards Recurrence of Grave Human Rights Violations-UN Report,' January 27, 2021.

85   Stephanie Nebehay and Alasdair Pal, 'Sri Lanka Faces U.N. Scrutiny Over Civil War Crimes,' Reuters, March 23, 2021.

86   International Commission of Jurists, 'Sri Lanka: Presidential Pardon of Former Army officer for Killing of Tamil Civilians is Unacceptable,' March 27, 2020.

87   Freedom House, 'Freedom in the World 2020: Sri Lanka', 2021.

88   Azzam Ameen, 'Sri Lankan Anthem Sung in Tamil for First Time Since 1949', BBC News, February 4, 2016.

89   High Commissioner of Human Rights, 'Sri Lanka on Alarming Path'.

90   Tamil Guardian, 'Who Cares, I Served My Country,'- Sri Lanka's Defence Secretary lashes out at UNHRC', February 26, 2021.

91   Meera Srinivasan, 'I Wish to Serve All Sri Lankans: Gotabaya', *The Hindu*, February 04, 2021.

92   Amnesty International, 'Justice reversed for victims of the Mirusuvil massacre, Sri Lanka', March 26, 2020.

93   International Commission of Jurists, 'Sri Lanka: Presidential Pardon'.

94   Ibid.

95   Anuradha Mittal, 'Endless War: The Destroyed Land, Life, and Identity of the Tamil People in Sri Lanka', The Oakland Institute (2021).

96   Ibid.

97   People for Equality and Relief in Lanka (PEARL), 'Militarisation of Government COVID-19 Response-OHCHR' (2020).

98   Andrea Malji, 'People Don't Want a Mosque Here: Destruction of Minority Religious Sites as a Strategy of Nationalism', *Journal of Religion and Violence*, 9, no. 1 (2021): 50–69.

99   Mittal, 'Endless War'.

100 DeVotta, 'The Genesis, Consolidation, and Consequences.'

101 Civil Society Groups Eastern Province, 'Sinhala 'Army & Archaeology' target 600 Sites for Heritage Occupation in Batticaloa' Report available at: www.tamilnet.com/art.html?catid=13&artid=39896.

102 Times of India, 'Tamil Memorial at Jaffna University Destroyed in Sri Lanka; Indian Leaders Express Shock', January 9, 2021.

103 BBC, 'Sri Lanka: Tamil War Monument to be Rebuilt after Hunger Strike', January 11, 2021.

104 Human Rights Watch, 'Sri Lanka: Due Process'.

105 Meera Srinivasan, 'Analysis | A Long March in Sri Lanka — to Register Protest, Forge a New Alliance', *The Hindu*, February 9, 2021.

106 International Truth and Justice Project, 'Sri Lanka: Torture and Sexual Violence by Security Forces 2020–2021' (2021).

107 Aanya Wipulasena and Mujib Mashal, 'Sri Lankan Minister Accused of Abusing Political Prisoners Resigns', *The New York Times*, September 15, 2021.

108 UNHRC, '46th session of the Human Rights Council'.

109 Human Rights Watch. "Sri Lanka: Police Abuses Surge Amid Covid-19 Pandemic," August 6, 2021.

110 Dong, Du, and Gardner, 'An Interactive Web-Based Dashboard'.

111 Al Jazeera, 'Sri Lanka Declares Food Emergency as Forex Crisis Worsens', August 31, 2021

5 Pakistan's Flailing Foreign Policy During Covid-19

Sahar Khan

Introduction

Covid-19 has wreaked havoc within South Asia, especially Pakistan. According to the World Health Organization, as of September 2021, there have been 1,232,595 confirmed cases of Covid-19 and 27,432 deaths associated with the virus.[1] The real numbers are probably higher. The number of coronavirus cases have also been increasing steadily as the Omicron variant has found its way to Pakistan. As at January 2022, Pakistan was experiencing a positivity rate of 3.66%. In other words, the daily cases were above 1,500.[2]

The Government of Pakistan, like all South Asian countries, has struggled to contain the virus. While Prime Minister Imran Khan was reluctant to fully close the economy immediately, his administration began to close the state's borders with Iran and Afghanistan as early as January 2020, which was followed by suspending all international flights, except from major airports (namely Islamabad, Karachi, and Lahore) by March.[3] March and April 2020 proved to be a critical time for Pakistan as the number of cases increased exponentially. The government eventually closed the border with China and temporarily halted China-Pakistan Economic Corridor (CPEC) projects; suspended the Pakistan Day parade (which was scheduled to be held on March 23, 2020) and all cricket matches; and began screening domestic travelers at the Jinnah airport in Karachi. President Arif Alvi tweeted that the public should avoid large gatherings and physical contact like hugging and shaking hands, especially if experiencing flu-like symptoms.[4] The National Security Council also met to discuss contact tracing and by the summer of 2020 established the National Command and Operation Center (NCOC) to coordinate the government's response to the pandemic.

The stress of COVID-19, therefore, added to pressures that the Khan administration was already experiencing since winning the election in 2018. After a year in office, Pakistan Tehreek-i-Insaf (PTI) unveiled its first annual budget for fiscal year 2019/20 and indicated a massive decline in its projected growth: from 6.2% to 2.4%.[5] To combat this downward trend, Prime Minister Khan announced the creation of a special commission to investigate

DOI: 10.4324/9781003248149-5

why the country was in so much debt. The Khan administration made increasing the sources of revenues (specifically those focused on establishing effective tax collection practices) and decreasing non-development expenditures a priority. In mid-2019 the International Monetary Fund (IMF) approved a $6 billion bailout package, but with strict conditions that had many government officials and economists predict that the aid package was too restrictive and unrealistic in its projections, especially as Pakistan's economy was shrinking instead of expanding.[6] When Covid-19 hit in early 2020, the economy was nowhere near improved, deepening concerns about an economic stagnation. Pakistan also remained on the Financial Action Task Force's (FATF)—a global money laundering and terrorist financing watchdog—"grey" list, which added to the country's economic and political pressures. CPEC was also slowing down, raising concerns that if the slowdown continued, it would negatively affect Pakistan's relationship with China. Finally, in 2019–20 Pakistan was also waiting to see what would become of the Afghan peace process, where the United States had a withdrawal date (May 1, 2021, according to deal between the Taliban and the United States), and the Afghan government and Taliban were at the negotiating table, but little progress was being made.

By the time the coronavirus took hold of Pakistan, in early 2020 it was clear that the Khan administration was in over its head, which tragically was the case with numerous countries worldwide. The government wasted no time in creating the NCOC, which is the joint civil-military task force, to coordinate the national Covid-19 response. The NCOC, however, is more military-led than civilian-led: high-ranking military officers play a visible role. While Khan chairs the meetings, especially those of the National Coordination Committee, which is the decision-making arm of the NCOC, Chief of Army Staff Qamar Bajwa also attends those meetings. In order to control the spread of the coronavirus, the NCOC imposed "smart lockdowns" across cities where numbers were increasing rapidly.[7] The Inter-Services Intelligence, Pakistan's premier intelligence agency, used its surveillance techniques for contact-tracing;[8] while effective, it has raised some concerns about how such a system of surveillance and tracking would continue to be used once the pandemic is over. When vaccines came out, Pakistan struggled to obtain them like most developing countries, but has acquired vaccines from China, Russia, and now the United States, and is steadily vaccinating its population.[9]

Granted, controlling the pandemic and preventing its spread, especially in an economically poor country like Pakistan, is a priority and the state should/must utilize all of its resources to combat the virus. Yet, the fact that the military has been at the forefront of what should be a civilian domain— responding to a health crisis—indicates just how deeply rooted the military is in Pakistan's society. While Pakistan's civil-military imbalance is old news—and not surprising when considering its political history (Jalal 2014; Jaffrelot 2015)—the deepening imbalance and reliance on the military has raised some eyebrows in both scholarly and academic circles. In this chapter,

I argue that this growing civil-military imbalance might, for once, work in Pakistan's favor, and allow it to refocus its flailing foreign policy on the country's economic concerns. I argue that the Covid-19 pandemic is a "critical interruption": a political event that does not necessarily threaten a state's self-identity needs, but forces a state to respond, and generate and regenerate narratives that legitimize and justify the state's policy choices, which eventually result in "institutionalized routines," which helps a state acquire ontological security.

To show this pivot, this chapter is divided as follows. The first section explains the concept of ontological security, arguing that the security achieved by meeting self-identity needs is equally important to a state's physical security. I also outline the factors that contribute to Pakistan's ontological security, and which ultimately impact its foreign policy. Finally, I will explain a generalizable ontological security framework I developed during my fieldwork in Pakistan, as a tool to better understand the state's identity and geostrategic needs. The second section dives into Pakistan's foreign policy, and the three main pillars that frame it, which are: it's acrimonious relationship with India, its weakening relationship with the United States, and its stable relationship with China. Pakistan's domestic response to Covid-19, however, has affected the country's foreign policy in unique ways, providing a rare opportunity for the state to reevaluate its foreign policy strategies and goals. The third section will provide pathways on how Pakistan can accomplish this shift toward equalizing its economic needs with its security ones, while remaining both physically and ontologically secure.

An Ontological Security Framework

The Concept of Ontological Security

What is ontological security? One of the core assumptions of realist international relations (IR) theory is that states prioritize their security and power—both of which are captured by a state's physical territory. The state's need for physical security—and its priority in protecting its physical territory—gives rise to the security dilemma and the practice of deterrence. The security dilemma is a core concept in IR theory: in an uncertain and anarchic international system in which states are rational actors, any action taken by a state to bolster its own security might threaten the security of another state, creating the classical dilemma. In a seminal essay, Jennifer Mitzen (2006) argues that states also prioritize their "ontological security" along with their physical security.

Ontological security refers to the security acquired by a continuous identity, and the agency that is created by maintaining this self-identity. The concept of ontological security—and seeking it—is drawn from the individual level, in which an individual seeks stability in an uncertain environment. Uncertainty at both the individual and state level is viewed as a threat. On the individual level, when an individual is uncertain of his/her actions and lacks confidence in their abilities to confront a problem, ontological *insecurity* is generated. Mitzen (2006) describes this state as "the deep, incapacitating state of not knowing which dangers to confront and which to ignore, i.e. how to get by in the world" (345). The individual then focuses on immediate, short-term needs, rather then focusing on planning for future needs and other long-term goals. When experiencing ontological insecurity, the individual is unable to realize a sense of agency. The rationalist perspective, however, assumes that all individual actors have sufficient information that allows them to act rationally. But uncertainty in the external environment reduces confidence. The mechanism for combating ontological insecurity lies in establishing routines via social relationships. Routines create stability and that stability helps to sustain identity. More importantly, the stability achieved by routines foster agency, leading to ontological *security*. Ontological security, therefore, is the condition in which an individual acquires confidence in his/her social relationships; the agency obtained by feeling ontologically secure allows to individual to hold on to their identity (Mitzen 2006, 345–48). Applied at the state level, a state acquires ontological security by creating routines via policies and relationships with other states via its foreign policy. By establishing and maintaining relationships with other states, a state reduces uncertainty, and hence creates its own agency. Ontological security, therefore, is similar to the state's need for physical security, and so like physical security, ontological security is a constant and cannot explain variation (Mitzen 2006, 343).

Mitzen (2006) presents three rationales for arguing that states seek ontological security. First, physical protection of a state is considered a priority and in IR, the state is considered a rational actor. The concept of sovereignty and its relationship to the physical body of the state, however, complicates the meaning of what is considered a state. Understanding a state's "personhood" encourages the development of looking beyond just physical security (Wendt 2004). Assuming that a state seeks both physical and ontological security, therefore, is conceptually compatible and "theoretically productive" (Mitzen 2006, 352). Second, each state is distinct: it consists of groups that prioritize maintaining their identity. Relationships between various groups lead to routines that reduce uncertainty and provide security and a collective national identity that allows for agency. It is logical then to assume that states are not just invested in protecting their physical body but also prioritize their identities and the factors that make them distinct in the international system. This also gives rise to the notion that state institutions have the ability to project images of the state—images that citizens become attached to and have complicated relationships with (Mitzen 2006, 352). For example, Brent Steele (2008) argues that states pursue moral, humanitarian, and honor-driven social actions to meet their self-identity needs even in instances where meeting such needs might compromise their physical security. The images and narratives that the state constructs, therefore, play an important role in a state's ontological security. The third rationale comes from empirical research: how sometimes applying micro-level assumptions and concepts allows for a better under-standing of macro-level outcomes and patterns. For example, there is a wide literature on American leaders during the Cold War and how each reacted similarly to the Soviet Union's actions despite themselves having very varied personalities (Mitzen 2006, 352; Dougherty and Pflatzgraff, Jr. 2001, 553–615). Ontological security, therefore, provides a sociological basis for understanding state actions (Mitzen 2006, 353).

An ontological security framework is a constructivist approach that is reflexive, and hence, can be interpretive in nature. Ontological security scholars do not use causal analysis to explain state behavior. Instead, we interpret state action by evaluating the political contexts that create social reality, recognizing that actions are not objective and devoid of context. As realists assume that leaders use political rhetoric to convince the public of "unsavory 'security' policies" (Steele 2008, 260), ontological security scholars assume that state agents use politics to secure the state's self-identity, use narratives to develop routinized foreign and domestic policies, promote a certain image of the state, and control the strategic environment in a way that reduces uncertainty (Steele 2008, 246–78). I conceptualize the processes of ontological security creation and main-tenance as an interconnected system in which state agents: 1) create a "biographical narrative" that employs a variety of narratives to create meanings and develop a state's self-identity needs; 2) determine "critical interruptions" that are political events that result in state action; and 3) legitimize continuous state policies, which I label as "institutionalized routines." By reconstructing state motivations, therefore, ontological security scholars are not only theorizing about state self-identity, but are also uncovering other avenues for understanding state rationality (Mitzen 2006; Steele 2008, 286–88).

Using an ontological security framework to analyze a state's foreign policy serves four important purposes. First, it forces scholars to rethink rationality and state rationale, which is often taken for granted in IR. Second, understanding how states seek ontological security helps to ana-lyze agency and discover new mechanisms by which a state practices and utilizes the agency it achieves by meeting its social and identity needs. As foreign policy is a key tool by which a state interacts with the interna-tional community, studying it using an ontological security framework is logical. Third, it unpacks the state, rather than black-boxing it, as is the traditional IR approach. Disaggregating the state and investigating how it maintains its ontological security is important for understanding state policies and actions, particularly with regards to its foreign policy. And finally, analyzing how a global event, like the Covid-19 pandemic, con-tributes to a state's ontological security provides the intellectual basis for problematizing foreign policy goals and national security interests: what they mean collectively and how they can respond to new threats.

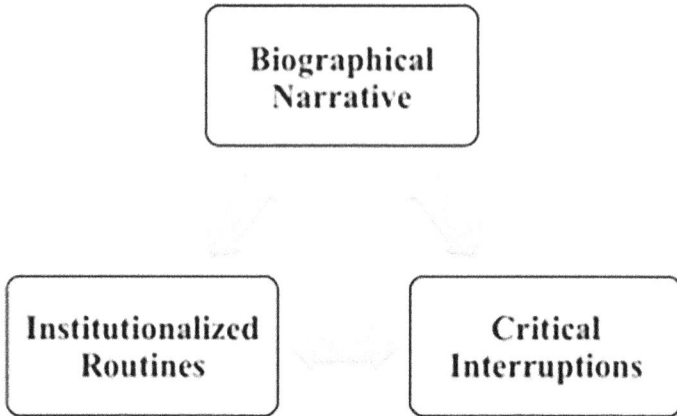

Figure 5.1 Processes of Ontological Security

Pakistan's Ontological Security: Seeking Stability via a Security-Focused Foreign Policy

The relationship between the state's actions and its identity is fluid: actions are dependent on identity while identity is reinforced by actions (Wendt 1992, 402–403).[10] For example, foreign policies need to assign meaning to a situation to be able to formulate a response, which utilizes specific identities of other states, regions, communities, and institutions (Hansen 2006, 6). Within an ontological security framework, identity-related needs are established through continuous actions, which fulfill the state's need for stability and certainty. An interruption in these actions causes instability and uncertainty, and hence leads to ontological *insecurity*. Identity, therefore, is not a standalone fact about a state. Instead, it needs to be interpreted in reference to state actions and inaction. This does not mean that I do not consider the history of the modern nation-state, as laid out by Richard Matthew (2002) or that I am not cognizant of the relationship between identity and nationalism. I use Lisa Wedeen's (2008) conception of nationalism. She argues that state institutions are critical to the development of nationalism because state institutions not only have the power to record, educate, and police the population, but are instrumental for tying together state sovereignty and the state's territory (7–8). In other words, state institutions reinforce the state's territory and borders while projecting and facilitating nationalist images and discourses. This is consistent with Lang's (2002) and Steele's (2008) argument that state agents constitute the state and the state's self-identity needs. I further their argument by positing that state agents use state institutions to form and drive the state's self-identity needs.

Neta Crawford (2002) puts forth three components of political identity: 1) a social identity, which refers to a sense of self in relation to and/or distinct from others, 2) a historical narrative about the self; and 3) an ideology (114). Pakistan's social identity is dominated by its security dilemma with India—a dilemma that has roots in the history of Muslim–Hindu tensions in the subcontinent (Gupta 1988, 112–118; Bose and Jalal 1997; Karim 2010; Wolpert 2010, 7–17). Indo–Pakistani tensions stem from six sources. First is Kashmir, the disputed territory that lies in the northeast of Pakistan, and over which the two states have fought three conventional wars and have had countless minor military exchanges (Wirsing 1993; Cohen 2002; Kapur 2010). The second is support of separatist movements across the border by each. India's support of the *Mukti Bahini*, Bengali freedom fighters, was crucial in the 1971 civil war that resulted in the breakup of Pakistan and formation of Bangladesh as a sovereign state (Dash 2008, 2139–2230; Ghoush 1989, 57–103). Pakistan's military strategy of supporting Kashmiri insurgent groups has provided Pakistan with a way to stealthily counter Indian rule in Kashmir while appeasing its own religious political parties, who often exploit the Kashmir dispute to mobilize public sentiment and increase their own legitimacy (Kapur and Ganguly 2012; Zahab and Roy 2004, 27; Byman 2005, 155–185). India claims that Pakistani-supported terrorist attacks within India have increased since 2002 (Byman 2005, 184)[11] while Pakistan denies the allegations. India also accuses Pakistan of lending support to the Sikh uprising in East Punjab (Hussain 1993, 153) that eventually resulted in the assassination of Prime Minister Indira Gandhi on October 31, 1984.

The third source of the Indo–Pakistani animosity is a military rivalry, which has resulted in both states developing nuclear weapons and missile capabilities (Ahmed 1999; Ganguly and Kapur 2010; Watt 2012; Chengappa 2016)—which almost led to a military conflict in Kargil in 1999 (Sagan and Waltz 2002; Rao 2016). The fourth source of tension has been the United States relationship with Pakistan. India views the US–Pakistani partnership as a hindrance and one that encourages Pakistan to challenge India regionally—this was especially the case during the Cold War (Ayoob 2000, 30; Muppidi 1999; Thornton 1993). Fifth is the religious and ethnic communal tensions aggravated by the Hindu nationalist Bharatiya Janata Party (BJP) of India (Buzan and Waever 2003, 108; Varshney 2002). The BJP does not seek separatism but instead seeks a strong national defense that includes nuclear deterrence. It also has a no-compromise policy on Kashmir and supports its integration into India via a special status granted to Kashmir in the Indian constitution. And the sixth source of Indo–Pakistani tension is water. The Indus Basin Irrigation System was originally conceived as a unified system, but it was split up after Partition. In April 1948 India cut off the water supply to Pakistan, resulting in an international water dispute between the two. A treaty was eventually signed in 1960 to resolve any future water disputes, but tensions often flare up, providing just another reason for both states to have a standoff (Kugelman 2016).

Pakistan's historical narrative is also intrinsically linked with Islam. The lack of consensus amongst South Asian Muslims on the meaning of Islam has created complicated and often competing conceptions of religion, identity, nationalism, and Muslim power in South Asia (Mullick and Yusuf 2009, 12). Pakistan not only inherited this puzzle but also unwittingly become a victim of the Two-Nation Theory, developed by Pakistan's founder, Mohammad Ali Jinnah. The Two-Nation Theory was a result of a combination of writings and speeches of Indian Muslim activists. It does not define "nation" on the basis of culture, language, history, territory, or customs but on religion. In the pre–Partition political environment, Jinnah and the Muslim League supported this theory that argued that Hindus and Muslims were two separate nations with distinct social orders, and hence, could never exist under a single, united nationality (Karim 2010). It remains unclear whether Jinnah wanted Pakistan to be a secular or a theocratic state (Jalal 1994; Karim 2010). Secularists, modernists, liberals, religious groups, etc. have all used Jinnah's philosophy to justify their own view of Pakistan, creating an ideological struggle within the country. As such, Pakistan's ideology is difficult to decipher. It is fraught with cultural contradictions and existential crises, and Pakistan still struggles with establishing a coherent identity (Cohen 2004; Shaikh 2009; Haider 2010; Wolpert 2010; Constable 2011; Jalal 2014; Shah 2014; Jaffrelot 2015; Rumi 2016).

What, then, is Pakistan's self-identity? It remains a puzzle as Pakistan is still developing a political identity. Two pillars, however, have emerged. The first is that Pakistan views itself as an "Islamic" country and a defender of Islam and protector of Muslims. The second pillar is that it must counter India, its hostile neighbor, and protect itself from Indian aggression and perceived anti-Islam stance. This second pillar feeds into Pakistan's foreign policy on the whole and has influenced the state's institutionalized routines, one of which is to prioritize its security concerns over its economic needs within its foreign policy.

A Rare Opportunity for Pakistan's Foreign Policy

Pakistan's Security-Focused Foreign Policy

Pakistan's foreign policy has three pillars: Its acrimonious relationship with India, its weakening relationship with the United States, and its stable relationship with China. The factors that drive Pakistan's relationship with India have been described above, but current tensions are based on the clash of the Khan and Modi administrations. Khan and the PTI was elected in 2018, while Modi and the BJP were re-elected in 2019. In August 2019, Prime

Minister Modi revoked the autonomous status of Jammu and Kashmir and Ladakh and implemented a wide variety of suppressive measures to deter Kashmiris from expressing their outrage. Pakistan and several other countries protested this move, but the Indian public welcomed it. The special status has not been reinstated.[12] The Modi administration also lobbied the FATF to put Pakistan on its grey list in 2018 and has been pushing to get the country on the black list, but has not succeeded. While Pakistan argues that India is using the non-political FATF for its political goals, India argues that it is simply trying to hold Pakistan accountable for being complicit in terrorist-related financing and money laundering.[13] Another current issue of contention between India and Pakistan is Pakistan's support of the Taliban, which has been ongoing since the 1990s (Rashid 2010).

Pakistan's support of the Taliban in Afghanistan has also deeply impacted its relationship with the United States over the past two decades. As the second pillar of Pakistan's security-focused foreign policy, the state's bilateral relationship with the United States is extremely important to it for a host of security, economic, and political reasons. Ever since the George W. Bush administration launched the Global War on Terror after the September 11, 2001 terror attacks on US soil, the bilateral relationship has been overly focused on counterterrorism and the US war in Afghanistan. After 20 years, the United States finally withdrew from Afghanistan, but the withdrawal has been a disaster. Throughout the war, the United States accused Pakistan of playing a "double game" (Coll 2018; Khan 2018) but also urged Pakistan to use its leverage with the Taliban to bring the group to the negotiating table. Now, the Taliban are back in power after the Afghan National Security Forces fell and President Ashraf Ghani and his cabinet fled the country. While no country has officially recognized the Taliban, Pakistan is urging the international community not to isolate the Taliban.[14]

The third pillar of Pakistan's foreign policy is its relationship with China. Pakistan and China have always had a steady relationship. Recently, China has supported bringing the Kashmir issue to the UN's agenda in its support of Pakistan.[15] Pakistan in turn has sided with China and opposed the interference of the UN Human Rights Council in China's domestic affairs, especially with respect to its treatment of Uyghurs.[16] CPEC, of course, has played a huge role in improving the bilateral relationship. As a developing country, Pakistan is in desperate need of infrastructure that CPEC projects provide. While it is unclear just how much CPEC has boosted industrial productivity and job creation, the various projects have put Pakistan on a path toward sustainable economic growth (Rafiq 2017).

These three pillars collectively have resulted in Pakistan creating a security-centric foreign policy; one that focuses—and prioritizes—its security interests over any other, such as economic interests. As a postcolonial state, Pakistan is hypersensitive about its territory, and became even more so after the 1971 war, which resulted in the creation of Bangladesh. Prioritizing physical security, however, is not a problem. Rather, it is a necessity. Yet,

Pakistan's prioritizing its physical security has led it to create a foreign policy that is too focused on its rivalry with India, too influenced by the United States, and too dependent on China. Above all, Pakistan's foreign policy puts security first, and its economy second, rather than on equal footing, which has ultimately led to the country practicing a foreign policy that reduces its ontological security. Covid-19, however, provides an opening to change this.

Covid-19 as a Critical Interruption

As described previously, a critical interruption is part of the process of a determining a state's ontological security. Critical interruptions are events that do not necessarily threaten a state's self-identity needs, yet they force states to respond, and generate and regenerate narratives that legitimize and justify the state's policy choices, which result in institutionalized routines. Some examples of critical interruptions are military coups, terrorist attacks, faulty elections, hurricanes, etc. While critical interruptions can be both predictable and unpredictable, they are always political. As the logic of ontological security dictates, the state's self-identity needs are constant—a state needs a stable identity to function in the world, just like a state needs to protect its territory to function in the international system. A critical interruption, therefore, disrupts state policies, forcing state agents to utilize the biographical narrative to respond through institutional changes, such as writing new legislation, creating specialized institutions and forces, eliminating an institution, reorganizing bureaucracy, and so on.

The state's ability to pursue ontological security is also dependent on how it deals with crises. Yet, not all crises are unpredictable, except rare environmental ones like tsunamis and earthquakes. As crises are social constructions, the time frames of when an event gets labeled "crisis" varies and depends on the actor. For example, the events that led up to the Cuban missile crisis, and the crisis itself, actually spanned a much longer period for both the Soviets and Cubans than it did for the Americans (Weldes 1999, 37–40). Second, not all crises threaten a state's self-identity or its routines. I argue that instead, crises "interrupt" routines, forcing state agents to manipulate state narratives to either create, alter, or end institutionalized routines via state institutions. Therefore, I use the label "critical interruptions." It is important to note that "critical interruptions" are not "critical junctures." Within historical and sociological institutionalism, "critical junctures" are defined as periods of significant change followed by a period of "path dependence" in which an institution follows a specific trajectory that is either maintained or reinforced over time (Pierson 2004, 54–78; George and Bennett 2005, 167; Gerring 2007, 2559–2560). The concept of critical junctures is employed in institutional analysis to uncover causality and examine structural (such as economic, cultural, ideological, organizational) influences on political action (Capoccia and Kelemen 2007). A critical interruption, however, is not concerned with causality in a strict, nomological sense, and cannot be studied as isolated incidents that affect institutions.

Critical interruptions are social constructions, and are intimately linked with the construction, reconstruction, and deconstruction of state identity. In this way, critical interruptions are more about the politics of practices and language of representation (Edelman 1988, 31). State agents are authorized to act on behalf of the state, and hence are responsible for acts that represent state actions. How state agents respond to crises and how crises affect state agents is co-constitutive: state identity can enable a critical interruption or conversely a critical interruption can enable state identity. Critical interruptions are not objective facts but rather political acts whose representation can be contested (Weldes 1999, 61).[17] For Weldes (1996) and Campbell (1998), state identity enabling a crisis is more logical because the subject is obvious: the anthropomorphized state subject produced in the foreign policy discourses of institutionalized states. This applies to critical interruptions as well. But how critical interruptions enable state identity varies from how Steele's (2008) "critical situations" enable state identity. In Steele's (2008) conceptualization, crises present a threat to a state's self-identity because they force state agents to take action and alter or end institutionalized routines (1284–1286). I argue that not all crises are threats, and so any changes made in institutionalized routines is not because of any danger associated with a threat. Rather, changes in institutionalized routines point to self-identity crises within the state over how the state constructs its self-identity needs, and consequently how the state views itself and wants to be viewed by others. Identities are constructed in relation to difference, where difference and identity are both fluid (Campbell 1998, 175–179). Identities are not necessarily constructed to counter threats or a different threatening Other (Campbell 1998, 232–235; Hansen 2006, 6–7).

Critical interruptions, however, are not just threats. Instead, they are significant events that enable and benefit state identity in three ways. First, they allow the state to claim sovereignty over their territory, and a monopoly of violence and the type of violence in the name of protecting that territory. By claiming to be the sole representative and/or sole protector of its population, the state reinforces itself within the international system. Second, critical interruptions allow the state agents to create institutions or structures of power that allow them—and by extension the state—to consolidate power internally (Tilly 1985, 171; Barnett 1992; Weldes 1999, 58). To do so, state agents use the state's narratives to legitimize and justify the state's consolidation of power over other actors within the state vying for power. Critical interruptions, therefore, are intrinsically related to the creation of a state's biographical narrative about self-identity, where the interaction of critical interruptions and narratives connects observable activities to policy responses. And third, critical interruptions allow for the articulation and rearticulation of the relationship between identity and difference as means to constitute and secure the state's self-identity (Weldes 1999, 58). I share

Campbell's (1998), Connolly's (1991), and Weldes's (1996, 1999) understanding of identity as always discursively constructed and produced in relationship with difference, where difference and identity are mutually constitutive. Hence, my conceptualization of critical interruptions takes into account the genealogy of identity within security studies, in which I am influenced by Michal Williams' (1998) argument. He asserts that debates within IR theory should not be between objectivist and positivist theoretical foundations. Instead, they should be more focused on the history of security studies and the politics surrounding theorizing security, which will highlight how identity—and difference—has been constructed to emphasize material power and create an objective foundation of analysis (Williams 1998).

Based on these criteria, as well as the politicization of the pandemic and Pakistan's subsequent response to Covid-19—creating the NCOC, using intelligence surveillance for contact-tracing, implementing "smart lockdowns," allowing mosques to remain open during Ramadan in 2020, etc.—indicate that the pandemic is a "critical interruption," and therefore, an opportunity for the state to make serious changes to its foreign policy. Furthermore, the politicization of Covid-19 is not just a phenomenon that Pakistan experienced, but one that is global in nature. In the case of Pakistan, the pandemic's politicization began when President Alvi agreed with religious leaders to keep mosques open during the month of Ramadan in 2020, despite the federal government issuing a nationwide lockdown.[18] So, mosques remained open and many prayed there, creating pockets where the virus could—and eventually—did spread. Civil society criticized the government for being weak on the lockdown, creating a clash between religious leaders and the general public. When vaccines were released, there was a great deal of misinformation and a poll released in January 2021 showed that 49% of Pakistanis did not want to get vaccinated.[19] Public awareness campaigns have helped, however.

Covid-19 as a Critical Interruption for Pakistan

The government of Pakistan responded as quickly as one would expect a developing country to respond. The timeline of major Covid-19-related events details the most significant actions of the government, but underlying these actions were two kinds of divisions: civil–military and socio-religious. While the socio-religious factors are important for understanding Pakistan's domestic policy and actions, the civil–military tensions provide a window into the country's foreign policy as well.

As described earlier, President Alvi's statements resulted in mosques remaining open during the second wave of the pandemic, creating dangerous pockets that eventually spread the disease. The Khan administration is scared of the religious right of Pakistan and the mob mentality. In Pakistan, no religious party has been able to win an election but in some ways it really doesn't need to because it has an unprecedented emotional hold on the people. The religious right…control the mob (Butt 2016). This is why

Table 5.1 Timeline of Major Covid-19 Events in Pakistan

	Event
January 2020	Balochistan and Gilgit-Balistan started taking precautionary measures to control the spread of Covid-19.
February 2020	Two cases of Covid-19 are confirmed in the beginning of the month. Closes border with China and Iran.
March 2020	Number of cases increase exponentially. All airports, except Islamabad, Lahore, and Karachi, are closed. Government announces a Rs. 1.2 trillion relief package for low-income groups. All provincial governments announced relief packages too.
April 2020	Number of cases keeps increasing. Government started its first lockdown, but mosques are reopened, leading to criticism regarding the government's mixed messages. State Bank of Pakistan introduces a temporary refinance scheme for businesses to deter layoffs.
May 2020	Government creates the National Command and Operation Center (NCOC) to coordinate its response. Federal government ends lockdown on May 9.
June 2020	Orders border with Afghanistan, allowing exports for the first time in three months.
July 2020	Trade relations with Afghanistan resume.
December 2020	Purchases 1.2 million doses of Covid-19 vaccine from China (called Sinopharm).
January 2021	China provides half a million vaccine does for free. Through COVAX, Pakistan received 17 million doses of the AstraZeneca vaccine.
March 2021	Lockdown is lifted on March 15.
May 2021	The Delta variant creates a spike in coronavirus cases in the state.

President Alvi's reluctance to close the mosques even during a pandemic was not possible as it ties into the country's "defender of Islam" mentality—and one of the primary ways it achieves ontological security.

The ways in which Pakistan's civil–military imbalance, however, become even more prominent during the pandemic does not just indicate how deep the imbalance is, but also provides a lens by which to reevaluate the country's foreign policy. For example, the formation of the NCOC in of itself is not odd, and neither is the fact that it is a joint institution, shared by the civilian and military sides. After all, several countries share bureaucracies. The NCOC's structure, however, indicates the power, prominence, and reliance on the military: instead of a chief minister or a federal health minister, the task of overseeing the coordination between federal and provincial governments was given to Commander of Army's Air Defense Command, Lt-Gen.

Hamood Uz Zaman Khan. What this means is that NCOC, which is tasked with optimizing information, decision-making related to Covid-19 and implementation of "smart lockdowns" to prevent the virus' spread, and which is supposed to serve as a liaison between the National Security Committee and the National Coordination Committee, falls under the care of the military.

In Pakistan's case, the pandemic highlighted several obvious and underlying political, social, and economic issues plaguing the country, as it did with almost every country. However, Covid-19 has also made Pakistani policymakers and the military leadership realize the importance of—and most significantly the need for—a strong economy. Without prioritizing the creation of a sustainable economy that is not dependent on IMF loans and developmental aid, Pakistan will remain insecure.

Toward a Non-Flailing Foreign Policy

Pivoting a foreign policy, and the geostrategic and national security interests that underlie it, is a Herculean task, and one that is rare and not easily achievable. Yet, it is not impossible. While Covid-19 and the lives it has claimed is a tragedy, it has also been a wake-up call for the world—and South Asia in particular. In South Asia, the pandemic has highlighted the weaknesses in government's public health systems, public mistrust with the government, the power of misinformation regarding public health and safety, and government's weak capacity in distributing vaccines. While most of these issues have been domestic-focused, all of these have also impacted each state's foreign policy. For Pakistan, the impact can be debated but one thing is clear: Covid-19 has provided Pakistan with the rare opportunity to make some series changes to its foreign policy.

There are three policies that Pakistan should invest in so that it can complete its foreign policy pivot; from a foreign policy that prioritizes security concerns over economic ones to where security and economy are tied together, ensuring that economic well-being and development adds to the state's physical and ontological security. The first pathway is to increase transparent revenue streams, which will create a better business environment and encourage foreign direct investments, and others. None of these can be done without eradicating external and fiscal imbalances. Before Covid-19, Pakistan had successfully started an economic reform program supported by the IMF and was able to continue the program during the pandemic. For example, Pakistan's foreign exchange buffers increased during mid-2019, which was the worst of the pandemic. The fiscal deficit actually fell as the pandemic ebbed. During the pandemic, instead of collapsing, Pakistan's banking institutions remained strong. For example, the Central Bank was able to provide significant economic stimulus packages, such as loan restructuring to borrowers to combat economic disruptions, loan extension programs to ease cash constraints on borrowers, and refinancing to prevent layoffs.[20] While Pakistan still needs an IMF program, it is on a slow and steady path of developing sustainable revenue streams.

The second pathway is to prioritize regional and economic development partnerships. On his latest trip to the United States, National Security Advisor Moeed Yusuf explained Pakistan's economic pivot and focus on "regional connectivity."[21] The aim of this strategy is for Pakistan to serve as a mediator—and to be viewed as a viable, reliable, and practical arbitrator by its neighbors. To do this, Pakistan's regional relationships must go beyond traditional security, such as defense contracts, weapons' systems and arms sales, and joint-military training (all of which are important) but more toward facilitating the movement of people and goods: opening borders, allowing tourism visas, creating intra-country transit systems, etc.[22]

The third pathway is to get off the FATF grey list—and stay off. One of Pakistan's biggest challenges has been combating money-laundering and effectively implementing anti-terrorist financing practices. Part of the problem is Pakistan's use of militant groups to counter India, especially Indian-administered Kashmir-based jihadi groups. India wants the international community to hold Pakistan accountable, and has used several international organizations to do so, with the FATF being one of them. Regardless of India's motivations, implementing all of FATF's recommendations and investing in an anti-money laundering and terrorism financing framework would help Pakistan both politically and economically. Politically, it would help the state improve its reputation while economically it will increase confidence in the state, which would ultimately attract all kinds of investments, potentially resulting in steady job growth that the country desperately needs. As of late 2021, Pakistan had completed 27 action points that the FATF requested.

None of these pathways are simple, and neither can they be done without careful analysis. Pakistan's policy in Afghanistan also threatens these pathways. After the US withdrawal and the Taliban's takeover of Afghanistan in August 2021, Pakistan has found itself in an advantageous position. Pakistan's alliance with the Taliban is not secret, even though the relationship has been deteriorating over the last two decades during the US war in Afghanistan. The Taliban have also evolved politically, though not ideologically. In the past, when the Taliban took over Kabul in 1996, the group was not really concerned with international recognition and legitimacy, which is not the case now. And this is where Pakistan finds itself as a mediator between the Taliban and the international community. The Khan administration have a friendly relationship with the Taliban, but since August 2021 the government has become more vocal about the international community working with the Taliban, while maintaining its official position of wanting a peaceful solution in Afghanistan. Yet, serving as a mediator between the Taliban and the world may be appealing to the Khan administration, it is a self-defeating long-term strategy for Pakistan. As an ally of the Taliban, Pakistan is actually in a position to hold the group accountable for its failed promises. Instead, Pakistan is again focusing on short-term security interests and basking in the moment where it's the main interlocutor in Afghanistan.

One thing is clear though: pivoting toward the economy and economic security will not only make Pakistan more physically secure, but will also make it more ontologically secure. Continuing to serve as a mediator between the Taliban and the world, however, will set Pakistan back to where it was: physically secure (perhaps) but ontologically insecure.

Conclusion

This chapter has used a novel approach to explain Pakistan's response to the Covid-19 pandemic, and the state's response. The ontological security framework, as outlined in this chapter, is based on the assumption that a state's ontological security is just as important and vital to its well-being as it's physical security. In other words, physical and ontological security are constants, and one that a state strives to achieve. Pakistan's ontological security is shaped by its relationship with India and Islam, both of which present the state with an existential crisis. These pillars of Pakistan's ontological security have resulted in the state having a foreign policy that has always prioritized its security needs over its economic ones, often creating a division between the two needs. Covid-19, however, has presented the state with a unique opportunity to pivot its foreign policy from a more security-centric one to an economic-centric one, where security and economic needs are equal. With this pivot in its foreign policy, Pakistan will be better positioned to secure itself physically and ontologically.

Notes

1   World Health Organization, https://covid19.who.int/region/emro/country/pk. Accessed on September 25, 2021.
2   Geo News, "Pakistan logs over 1,000 COVID-19 cases for fifth straight day," January 10, 2022, www.geo.tv/latest/392541-pakistan-logs-over-1000-cases-for-fifth-straight-day.
3   SAMAA, "Number of coronavirus cases in Pakistan jumps to 28: officials," March 13, 2020, www.samaa.tv/living/health/2020/03/number-of-coronavirus-cases-in-pakistan-jumps-to-28-officials.
4   Arif Alvi, Twitter, March 12, 2020, https://twitter.com/ArifAlvi/status/1238288917658587138.
5   Hufsa Chaudhry, "Budget 2020: Govt predicts 2.4pc growth, Rs7 trillion in expenditures," *Dawn*, June 12, 2019, www.dawn.com/news/1484102.
6   Kunwar Khuldune Shahid, "The IMF Takeover of Pakistan," *The Diplomat*, July 18, 2019, https://thediplomat.com/2019/07/the-imf-takeover-of-pakistan.
7   Library of Congress, "Pakistan: 'Smart Lockdown' Imposed across Cities of Pakistan as Covid-19 Cases Grow Rapidly," June 25, 2020, www.loc.gov/item/global-legal-monitor/2020-06-25/pakistan-smart-lockdown-imposed-across-cities-of-pakistan-as-covid-19-cases-grow-rapidly.
8   See Niha Dagia and Niha Dagia, "Inside Pakistan's COVID-19 Contact Tracing," *The Diplomat*, July 1, 2020, https://thediplomat.com/2020/07/inside-pakistans-covid-19-contact-tracing and Asad Hashim, "Pakistan using intelligence services to track coronavirus cases," Al Jazeera English, April 24, 2020, www.aljazeera.com/news/2020/4/24/pakistan-using-intelligence-services-to-track-coronavirus-cases.

9 Saeed Shah and Waqar Gillani, "In Pakistan, Saying 'No' to Covid-19 Vaccine Carries Consequences," *Wall Street Journal*, June 22, 2021, www.wsj.com/articles/ saying-no-to-covid-19-vaccine-in-pakistan-carries-consequences-11624359601. Also see this Reuters tracker for daily updates: https://graphics.reuters.com/world-cor onavirus-tracker-and-maps/countries-and-territories/pakistan.

10 For an analysis and genealogy of "identity" within security studies, see Williams 1998.

11 Some examples of attacks where India has accused Pakistan are: 1) American cultural center in Kolkata on January 22, 2002; 2) in Kaluchak on May 14, 2002; and 3) on the Ram temple in Ayodhya on July 5, 2005 (attackers are believed to belong to Lashkar-e-Taiba); on military camp in Uri, near the Line of Control that divides Kashmir between India and Pakistan on September 19, 2016.

12 See Anchal Vohra, "Modi Took Complete Control of Kashmir 2 Years Ago— and Got Away with It," *Foreign Policy*, August 3, 2021, https://foreignpolicy.com/ 2021/08/03/modi-took-control-of-kashmir-2-years-ago-and-got-away-with-it/ and BBC World, "Viewpoint: Why Modi's Kashmir move is widely supported in India," August 15, 2019, www.bbc.com/news/world-asia-india-49354697.

13 See Dipanjan Roy Chaudhury, "India will lobby to put Pakistan on FATF blacklist at Paris meet," *The Economic Times*, February 18, 2019, https://econom ictimes.indiatimes.com/news/politics-and-nation/india-will-lobby-to-put-pakista n-on-fatf-blacklist-at-paris-meet/articleshow/68041049.cms and Naveed Siddiqui, "India's admission on FATF politization vindicates Pakistan's stance: FO," *Dawn*, July 19, 2021, www.dawn.com/news/1635854/indias-admission-on-fatf-politicisa tion-vindicates-pakistans-stance-fo.

14 Edith M. Lederer, "The AP Interview: Don't Isolate the Taliban, Pakistan Urges," Associated Press, September 23, 2021, https://apnews.com/article/pakistan-afghanista n-united-nations-taliban-shah-mehmood-qureshi-258c17303271aa440cf60f5a9444e143.

15 Shi Jiangtao, "China puts Kashmir on United Nations agenda to boost isolated Paki-stan's cause," *South China Morning Post*, August 16, 2019, www.scmp.com/news/china/ diplomacy/article/3023184/china-puts-kashmir-united-nations-agenda-boost-isolated.

16 *Global Times*, "65 Countries express opposition to interference in China's internal affairs at UN Human Rights Council," September 25, 2021, www.globaltimes. cn/page/202109/1235032.shtml.

17 I have used "environmental disaster" as an illustration of a critical interruption. While natural disasters do not start off as political acts, their politicization is dependent on the states' response and representation of the disaster. For exam-ple, Bangladesh's response to Cyclone Marion in 1991, the effect of the 2004 tsunami on conflicts in Sri Lanka and Indonesia, Pakistan's response to the 2005 earthquake in Azad Kashmir, and the US response to the *Deepwater Horizon* oil spill in the Gulf of Mexico in April 2010, are all examples of natural disasters that became political as aid efforts and disaster management challenged various aspects of state sovereignty. In an ontological security framework, therefore, they have the potential to serve as critical interruptions.

18 International Crisis Group. "Pakistan's COVID-19 Crisis." Briefing No. 162. August 6, 2020. www.crisisgroup.org/asia/south-asia/pakistan/b162-pakistans-covid-19-crisis.

19 Diaa Hadid. "Pakistan's Vaccine Worries: Rich People and Conspiracy Theor-ists." Goats and Soda. NPR. January 29, 2021. www.npr.org/sections/goatsa ndsoda/2021/01/29/961258106/pakistans-vaccine-worries-rich-people-and-conspira cy-theorists.

20 United States Institute of Peace, "Pakistan's Economic Future: A Conversation with Pakistani Finance Minister Shaukat Tarin on Economic Stability, Pakistan's Regional Role, and Geoeconomics," October 13, 2021, www.usip.org/events/pa kistans-economic-future.

21 United States Institute of Peace, "Pakistan's National Security Outlook: A Conversation with Pakistani National Security Advisory Moeed Yusuf," August 5, 2021, www.usip.org/events/pakistans-national-security-outlook.
22 See Sahar Khan, "The Untapped Economic Potential of the Pakistan-Turkey Relationship," *South Asian Voices*, April 20, 2021, https://southasianvoices.org/the-untapped-economic-potential-of-the-pakistan-turkey-relationship.

References

Butt, Ahsan. "Street Power: Friday Prayers, Islamist Protests, and Islamization in Pakistan." *Politics and Religion*, 9, no. 1 (March 2016): 1–28.

Coll, Steve. *Directorate S: The C.I.A. and America's Secret Wars in Afghanistan and Pakistan*. New York: Penguin Press, 2018.

Connolly, William. *Identity/Difference: Democratic Negotiations of Political Paradox*. Ithaca: Cornell University Press, 1991.

Crawford, Neta C. "The Passion of World Politics: Propositions on Emotion and Emotional Relationships." *International Security*, 24, no. 4 (Spring 2000): 116–156.

Dougherty, James E., and Pfaltzgraff, Jr., Robert L. *Contending Theories of International Relations: A Comprehensive Survey*. 5th Edition. New York: Longman, 2001.

Hansen, Lene. *Security as Practice: Discourse Analysis and the Bosnian War*. Kindle Edition. London: Routledge, 2006.

Jaffrelot, Christophe. *The Pakistan Paradox: Instability and Resilience*. Kindle Edition. Oxford: Oxford University Press, 2015.

Jalal, Ayesha. *The Struggle for Pakistan: A Muslim Homeland and Global Politics*. Kindle Edition. Cambridge, MA: Harvard University Press, 2014.

Khan, Sahar. "*Double Game: Why Pakistan Supports Militants and Resists U.S. Pressure to Stop*." *Policy Analysis*, No. 849, Cato Institute. September 20, 2018. www.cato.org/policy-analysis/double-game-why-pakistan-supports-militants-resists-us-pressure-stop.

Lang, Anthony F. "The Politics of Punishing Terrorists." *Ethics and International Affairs*, 24, (Spring 2010): 3–12.

Mitzen, Jennifer. "Ontological Security in World Politics: State Identity and the Security Dilemma." *European Journal of International Relations*, 12, no. 3 (2006): 341–370.

Rafiq, Asif. "*The China-Pakstan Economic Corridor: Barrier and Impact*." USIP Peaceworks, United States Institute of Peace. October 25, 2017. www.usip.org/publications/2017/10/china-pakistan-economic-corridor.

Rashid, Ahmed. *Taliban: Militant Iskam, Oil and Fundamentalism in Central Asia*. Second Edition. New Haven: Yale University Press, 2010.

Steele, Brent J. *Ontological Security in International Relations: Self-Identity and the IR State*. New York: Routledge, 2008.

Wedeen, Lisa. *Peripheral Visions*. Kindle Edition. Chicago: Chicago University Press, 2008.

Weldes, Jutta. "Constructing National Interests." *European Journal of International Relations*, 2, no. 3 (1996): 275–318.

Wendt, Alexander. *Social Theory of International Relations*. Cambridge, UK: Cambridge University Press, 1999.

6 Covid-19 in Nepal and the Existential Predicaments of Poverty and Governance

Shiva Raj Mishra and Bipin Adhikari

Introduction

The Covid-19 pandemic has proven to be a major catastrophe globally, which is leaving an indelible scar on the history of humankind. Although the impact from Covid-19 was indiscriminate, low-income, and middle-income countries were particularly affected because of fragile health systems, poor infrastructure, and lack of preparedness (Shrestha et al. 2021). Nepal is a low-income country in South Asia, sandwiched between China and India. The ongoing Covid-19 pandemic has already become a disaster on the proportions of the recent Gorkha earthquakes in 2015 (Adhikari et al. 2017, Adhikar et al. 2020). By the time this chapter was written, the Covid-19 pandemic infected nearly 700,000 individuals (230 per 100,000 population) and caused nearly 10,000 deaths in Nepal (3.3 per 100,000 population) (Ministry of Health and Population, Nepal 2021). In terms of sheer numbers, the Covid-19 pandemic has surpassed the reported 9,000 deaths by 2015 Gorkha earthquakes (Adhikari et al. 2016, Adhikari et al. 2020). In addition, the lockdown measures implemented following the Covid-19 pandemic has severely affected the economy, health service delivery and utilization; mostly affecting population from poor households (Adhikari et al. 2020, Singh et al. 2020, Singh et al. 2021).

The pandemic has come during a time of political flux. Nepal is among the youngest federal democratic republics, having its century old monarchy end in 2006 through democratic movement and peace accord with rebel forces in 2006. Despite these ostensible political milestones, the country is immersed in major systemic problems such as poverty, poor accountability and corruption affecting public sectors (Figure 6.1), which combined together might affect the performance of Nepal's new federal architecture (Adhikari et al. 2020). Nepal also witnessed a massive economic and political storm that ranged from shrinking international aid to a faltering relationship with India, all of which have added woes to its lagging developmental efforts post-earthquakes (Adhikari et al. 2017, Adhikari et al. 2020). The new political structure itself has been tested repeatedly, the outcomes of which have shown that the overall health

DOI: 10.4324/9781003248149-6

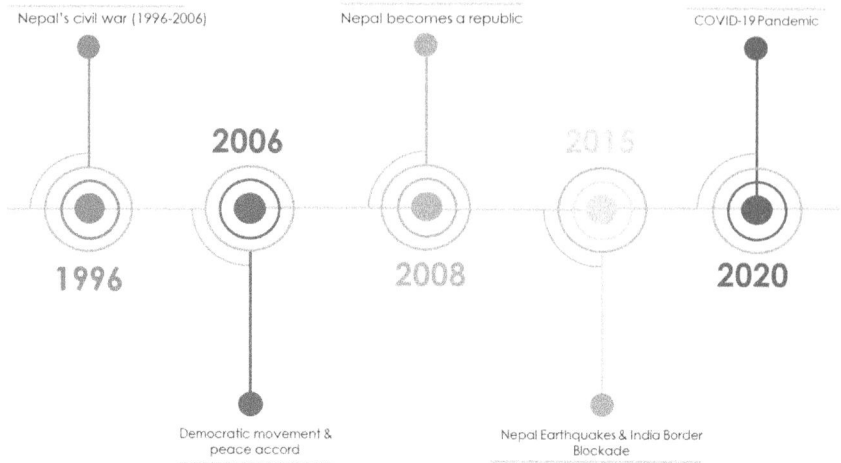

Figure 6.1 Putting Nepal's Covid-19 pandemic in the context of socioeconomic and political changes over the past 20 years
Adapted from author's prior work (Adhikari et al. 2020).

system is severely constricted by lack of budgetary capacity to mobilize resources at the local level both for Covid-19 response as well as other developmental activities (Shrestha et al. 2021). The seven federal provinces and 753 municipalities are lagging in enacting laws, mobilizing resources, and taking pre-emptive efforts to halt the spread of the pandemic, which has been especially prominent in rural and remote populations (Shrestha et al. 2021). Surpassing the impact of the earthquakes, the Covid-19 pandemic could reignite and widen the social inequalities.

Ending ten years of conflict, Nepal signed a peace accord with rebel forces in 2006 leading a new political wave in the country. Country abolished the monarchy in 2006, became the federal democratic republic of Nepal. Two massive earthquakes rattled Nepal in 2015, followed by India's economic blockade severely paralysing the country's health and economy. The Covid-19 pandemic has further increased Nepal's woes.

Here in this chapter, we discuss Nepal's response to Covid-19 based on social, ethnographic, and political examination. The chapter is divided into four sections. First, we offer a narrative account of Nepal's response to the Covid-19 pandemic, starting from the detection of the first case in the country. The second section discusses the health system response in the wake of Covid-19 infection and rapid transmission across the country. The third section discusses the impact of the pandemic on health, the economy, and development. The final section discusses the possible lessons from the pandemic for future preparedness.

When Covid-19 Hit a Himalayan Nation

Nepal's first Covid-19 infection was reported in a 32-year-old student returnee from the Wuhan University of Technology in China on January 3, 2020 (Bastola et al. 2020, Pokharel et al. 2020). He presented with minor symptoms and after thirteen days in the hospital, made a full recovery. With the successful identification and management of its first case, the country implemented a series of activities to boost the Covid-19 preparedness (Adhikari et al. 2020). Under the leadership of the Ministry of Health and Population, monitoring and health desks teams were set up at the major border checkpoints and locations around the country including country's only international airport in Kathmandu (Pokharel et al. 2021, Nepal 2021, Rayamajhee, et al. 2021). In the absence of testing facilities, prevention activities in the initial days were limited to screening for fever and cough. In the subsequent weeks, a network of hub and satellite hospitals were established (Adhikari et al. 2020, Shrestha et al. 2021). Personal protective equipment was distributed. And, within a month of reporting the first case, the first confirmatory PCR test were run from January 27 2020 (Bastola et al. 2020, Pokharel et al. 2020).

Nepal has had previous experiences with epidemics as well as natural disasters, including the recent earthquakes (Adhikari et al. 2016, Adhikari et al. 2017, Shrestha et al. 2021). These experiences, together with the political changes and general instability, has forged Nepal's resilience towards both disease epidemic and natural disasters (Adhikari et al. 2017). Nonetheless, Covid-19 has been a unique global burden that tested the country's health system's capacity to deal with its consequences (El Bcheraoui et al. 2020, Pokharel et al. 2020). As a result, Covid-19 became a global common test for countries fighting off the pandemic. Thus, how global, regional, and national level efforts were made against the pandemic are worthwhile to reflect and learn from which can ultimately help for future pandemic preparedness (El Bcheraoui et al. 2020, Pokharel et al. 2020).

The early inferences that some nations and regions were spared from the Covid-19 pandemic were simply proven to be untrue (Etienne et al. 2020, *The New York Times* 2020, United Nations 2020). Even the nations that were praised for their apt handling of the pandemic later got overwhelmed equally if not more compared to regional comparators (European Commission 2020). For instance, Germany, Singapore, Taiwan, South Korea, and New Zealand did relatively well in the initial pandemic response, although their achievements were soon challenged by resurgence of cases (The Wall Street Journal 2021). The fluidity and unpredictability of the Covid-19 pandemic soon became a hallmark characteristic, which added a layer of complexity for researchers, policymakers, stakeholders and the public. The spread of the Delta variant from the Indian sub-continent to Southeast Asian countries remarkably demonstrated the unavoidability of remaining as an island nation or an isolated state. Nations across the region that shared borders were a conduit/and a transmission path for Covid-19 and again leaves a strong message that no countries can absolutely be isolated even if borders were politically sealed (European Commission 2020). This was also evident from the spread of the Delta variant in Wuhan where the control measures for the initial epidemic was deemed to be successful. Inability to fight against Covid-19 as an isolated state further reiterates the notion of seeing health as a global entity that should be gazed through the notion of regionalism and cosmopolitanism. Such a notion has been increasingly gaining traction as more countries have realized that 'No-one is safe until everyone is safe' and applies for current spread of Delta variant and vaccination coverage (UNICEF 2021).

Interconnectedness of the nations within the region and outside warrants a redefinition of global health that should call for a globally collaborated efforts towards the pandemic (World Health Organisation 2021). Lacking collaborative and concerted efforts in fighting against the pandemic was one of the major drivers of uncontrolled pandemic. Thus, solidarity and call for concerted efforts between nations and regions are critical in a fight against the pandemic. While this strengthens the central tenet of globalization in health and disease outbreak, national disease preparedness and the characteristics of health system are unique and critical to learn and adapt for the future preparedness (Shrestha et al. 2021). The sub-section below describes Nepal's unique encounter with Covid-19, health system response and lessons for future disease outbreak.

Covid-19 Preparedness and Response: Feeble and Lackadaisical

Nepal's response to the Covid-19 pandemic is filled with a series of half-hearted steps mostly arising from political misalignment between central and local governments and widespread corruption impeding efficiency of activities in the ground (Mishra and Adhikari 2019, Adhikari et al. 2020, Adhikari et al. 2020). The pandemic was followed by a leadership vacuum, due to repeated transfers of staff, crippling efforts to keep the public safe. Interestingly, the country did not have, then nor does even today a Covid-19 response and exit plan – leading to misalignment of goals between central and local governments (Shrestha et al. 2021). Lacking coordination and resources to surmount the pandemic, Nepal's response to the Covid-19 pandemic is seemingly feeble and lackadaisical.

Nepal's Covid-19 response has been widely documented in a series of publications including in our own works, detailing every facet of public health response: mismanagement of resources, corruption, and leadership failures (Mishra and Adhikari 2019, Ministry of Health and Population, Nepal 2021). Poor handling of the pandemic was criticized widely and echoed with the previous handling of natural disasters, particularly the Gorkha earthquakes (Shrestha et al. 2021). While Gorkha earthquakes were standalone tests for Nepal's health system and its preparedness, Covid-19 was a global health problem that swept through the open borders and echoed the epidemic curves of India (Adhikari et al. 2020). If we take a proximal look at Nepal's response to Covid-19, we cannot extricate the geopolitical interconnectedness of the region, particularly how Nepal shares around 1,600 km with India on the east, west and the south (Adhikari et al. 2020). Understanding length of border alone with India as a determinant of pandemic in Nepal would be an understatement unless we account the geographical characteristics that describes the nature of border crossings, population density, cultural similarities, trade, and many other factors.

For instance, Nepal's southern borders are much more connected to India than the northern border to China (Bansh Jha 2013). What connects more to India is not just the geographical landscape that much of it has plane terrain but it is the population density on either side of the border that are high which conduces frequent border crossings (Singh 2010). In the northern border with China, the geographical landscape is hostile, a lot of which are uncrossable, owing to high mountains, rough terrain, cold weather, snow, and high altitudes. In addition, the population density on the either side of the northern border is low thus the population movement, cultural exchange and trade are slimmer (Singh 2010, DW 2021). These border conditions pose a huge implication for disease epidemiology (Rijal et al. 2018, Adhikari et al. 2020). For instance, historical and current malaria epidemiology is heavily affected by migrants returning Nepalese laborers from India where Nepal's malaria elimination strategy simply focuses on how to tackle the importation of malaria from India (Rijal et al. 2018). More than 50% of malaria cases in Nepal are imported from India. Similarly, the first case of dengue which was detected in a Japanese tourist who came from India, now cases of dengue ascend the Himalayan altitudes pushing the boundary further north annually (Rijal et al. 2021).

Thus, disease epidemiology corresponds with the population movement across the border (Smith et al. 2019). A large portion of Nepalese population is dependent on the Indian economy, that is, India has been the main destination for both skilled and unskilled workers who earn money and remit to Nepal (Rijal et al. 2018, Smith et al. 2019). Such an interdependence explains how these population when they return to Nepal during annual leave or festivals tend to carry the diseases with them. Another important disease that is inextricably linked with labor/unskilled population is HIV/AIDS (Poudel et al. 2004, Nepal 2007, Vaidya and Wu 2011). Much of the unskilled population in Nepal is either lured by economic opportunities or are trafficked to India who ultimately get succumbed to all sorts of jobs including prostitution, unsecured sex and inevitably carry such chronic conditions that require lifelong treatment (Poudel et al. 2004, Awasthi et al. 2015).

Taking a wider and more detailed geopolitical perspective, it is not surprising to see the Covid-19 pandemic echoing the disease curves of India. Nepal's Covid-19 surge echoed the Indian curve so much that the disease was an additional list among the existing diseases that require cross border collaboration for elimination (e.g. Malaria). (Adhikari et al. 2020). Nonetheless, Nepal's leaders failed to anticipate the epidemic outbreak of India and make efforts to prevent outpouring of cases from the border. Unfortunately, Nepal was not prepared to absorb the impact. There are several reasons why Nepal could not withstand the Covid-19 pandemic from southern border.

Although Nepalese leaders anticipated that Covid-19 cases could enter from international borders, having a high density of population movement across the border overwhelmed the public health measures such as fever screening check-posts at the border, and quarantine centers (Pokharel et al. 2021). Population pressure at the international borders was not unique to Nepal although the characteristics of border and its porosity are unique and requires a tailored approach. While geo-political context offers valuable insights around how Covid-19 echoed the history of other diseases, inspecting at the core elements of health system preparedness is paramount in understanding and forging lessons for the future (Shrestha et al. 2021).

Prior to the pandemic, Nepal had a total of 26,930 hospital beds (8.97 per 100,000 population), 1,595 ICU beds (0.53 per 100,000), 840 ventilators (0.28 per 100,000), and 194 hospitals with ICU facilities (0.06 per 100,000) (Ministry of Health and Population, Nepal 2020). There is a critical shortage of health providers: doctors, nurses and midwives. There were only 67 health workers (doctors, nurses, or midwives) per 100,000 population and 17 doctors per 100,000 population exists for the entire country, while only 40% of them work in rural areas, depriving access to basic and specialist health services (Tamang et al. 2020). When the pandemic hit the country, it triggered a significant exodus of the health workforce: increased absenteeism, voluntary termination and transfers adding further complexity to a constrained presence of health workers in rural areas.

Health system preparedness builds on the mantra of preventive medicine: "prevention is better than a cure" and "over-preparedness is better than under-preparedness." Nonetheless, investment in pre-emptive public health measures is often neglected and overlooked in Nepal where clinical care and public health measures are often reactive (Shrestha et al. 2021). Likewise, reactive measures in public health are often a hallmark characteristic of health systems where resources are often constrained to deliberate for the proactive and preventive measures. However, attributing to constrained resources alone for poor preventive measures would be an excuse as few developing nations with strong motivation for preparedness have dealt the pandemic well (Conversation 2020). For instance, Bhutan, Maldives, and Sri Lanka have excelled in adopting measures that were necessary to ensure that the health system had adequate preparedness to deal with the pandemic (Amaratunga et al. 2020, Sarkar et al. 2020). What lies at the heart of the preparedness is the motivation to invest in something that might look intangible in the immediate future but bears significant implications for long term future, and sometimes, resources that are invested for preparedness might never really be utilized. Nevertheless, having the resources in place regardless of how they might (might not) be utilized, characterizes the essence of 'preparedness.' Much of the measures taken during the Covid-19 pandemic in Nepal were rolled out once the cases started surging where initial few cases were simply underestimated and overlooked. The benefits of preparedness were overlooked and the price for the under-preparedness was simply beyond anticipation.

The health system of Nepal bears characteristics that echo with fragile and weak health systems in most of the developing countries. Although Nepal's state-run public health services are mostly affordable, their accessibility and quality of care are questionable, particularly as parallel running private sectors tend to excel in offering quality care (Ghimire et al. 2020). Major proportion of public health care services are accessed through out-of-pocket money although government health insurance coverage is gradually increasing over the last few years (Mishra et al. 2015). The Nepal's private sector is responsible for nearly 70% of all health expenditures, of which a majority of the cost (~80%) is paid out-of-pocket (Mishra et al. 2015). Another characteristic feature of Nepal's health system is that health services, including both public and private operations, are urban centric: only 59% of households have access to health services within 30 minutes in rural areas compared to 86% of households in urban areas (Adhikari and Mishra 2016, Adhikari et al. 2017). On average, it takes nearly 135 minutes for the rural population to reach their nearest health facility (e.g. health posts); which they make these journeys via cycle/transport (40%) and walking-only (50%) (Ashworth et al. 2019). The lack of motorized transport and the difficult topography is responsible for delays in seeking health services which combined with the individual's inability to pay in a highly privatized health sector severely compromises individual's ability to access health services when and where it is needed. In addition to these existing caveats of the health system, transition into a federal health system based on the new constitution, is fraught with many issues: from lacking clear demarcation of roles and responsibilities between the federal, provincial, and local governments, lack of human, material and financial resources and a widespread corruption impeding deployment of capable frontline health workers (Ghimire et al. 2020). The existing challenges will continue to pose threat to post-Covid-19 plans affecting delivery of essential health services.

Although Nepal anticipated the Covid-19 pandemic, health system preparedness was sluggish and lackadaisical, particularly as the race against the pandemic was at first started delayed and second, coordination between the tiers of governance structure was poor (Shrestha et al. 2021). The other chronic problem that has crippled Nepal's health system is lack of adequate health human resources, more prominently at the provincial and local levels. While the provincial and local level structures were meant to be independent enough to take on roles and responsibilities, they were simply unable to undertake the responsibilities because of these existing challenges. One of the less pronounced challenges during Covid-19 was also the characteristics of the disease that was highly contagious, and Nepal did not have a specialized pandemic response team, or infectious disease handling team (Pokharel et al. 2020). The lack of specialist teams also impeded the adoption of protocols and guidelines for effective management. The development of a protocol, and treatment guidelines consumed significant time while Covid-19 was overbearing on frontline health workers. Preparing good reports, guidelines and proto-cols, instead of focusing on operationalization and implementation of Covid-19 preparation and care demonstrates characteristics of 'paper tigers,' which can offer complacency and false sense of achievements. The remaining amount of time and resources required to tackle the disease simply constrained Nepal's health system. The severity scores of respiratory compli-cations, due to Covid-19-required intensive care units with resources for respiratory support such as ventilators which was also in chronic shortage in Nepal (Pokharel et al. 2020, Shrestha et al. 2021).

Establishing Covid-19-specific hospitals and quarantine centers were some of the illustrative preparedness measures taken. Nonetheless, lack of resources, both equipment, human resources and importantly ICUs loomed as major gaps in both preparedness and management of the cases (Pokharel et al. 2020, Shrestha et al. 2021). These gaps were multiplied, owing to poor governance, and coordination between various tiers of government. Because of these gaps and coordination/governance failures, Nepal had to utilize lock down as an intervention rather than a mere strategy to provide more time to build up the interventions such as establishing hospitals. For instance, lock down could have been used as tracing the cases, surveillance and isolating the population in a targeted manner. Instead, lockdown became a source of complacency because of its ostensible impact in reducing the number of cases (Singh et al. 2020). Although concerns started arising, due to prolonged lockdowns, such as their impact on other health conditions (routine immu-nization), economy and development related works (Singh et al. 2020, Singh et al. 2021).

Impact on Health, the Economy, and Development

The Covid-19 pandemic had a noticeable impact on three areas: health, econ-omy, and development (Rayamajhee et al. 2021, Singh et al. 2021). Although these broad areas are interlinked, it is essential to analyze and extricate how the pandemic affected each of the areas. An analysis into these three areas can highlight how health as a concern transcends and impacts an individual and its meso- (e.g., household/community's economy and wellbeing) and macro-spheres (e.g., development of advanced health care facilities). At the same time, it is critical to understand that these meso- and macro-spheres directly and indirectly affect the human health. Series of reports that came out during the early phase of pandemic showed that significant disruption and delays in health services due to lockdowns, increased worries, and anxiety of Covid-19, and lack of information and awareness contributed to rapid spread of pandemic

(Pokharel et al. 2021, Rayamajhee et al. 2021). These studies reported lack of availability and access to testing facilities, isolation, and quarantine centers due to disruption in transportation services (Singh et al. 2020, Rayamajhee et al. 2021, Singh et al. 2021).

There are only a handful of studies that have documented the impact of service disruption on health (Singh et al. 2020, Rayamajhee et al. 2021, Singh et al. 2021). The widespread fear owing to transmissibility, severity and the scores of deaths drew all attention towards Covid-19, increasingly referred to as 'covidization' in the literature in global health (Pai 2020). Inevitably, this had a major impact on health services for other health conditions. Because of major focus and prioritization on Covid-19 cases that also entailed turning all or parts of health care institutions into Covid-19 care institutions, in fact impeded the health services for other health conditions. Routine health care through outpatient-departments were put on hold and these affected most of the non-Covid-19 health conditions (Sharma et al. 2021). Both academic and non-academic reports started to emerge around how lack of antenatal care for pregnant mothers affected their attendance including increase in morbidity and mortality associated with the other diseases (Gurung et al. 2020, Singh et al. 2021).

Routine vaccinations were also affected by the Covid-19 pandemic, to an extent that there were reports of measles outbreak from various regions of Nepal (*Nepali Times* 2020). Impediments in routine vaccination due to Covid-19 echoed across the region and countries (UNICEF 2020). In developing countries where health services are already constrained by plethoric reasons, delayed health seeking behavior, or its absence takes a heavy toll on morbidity and mortality (Adhikari et al. 2019, Marahatta et al. 2020). In such an existing context, Covid-19 disrupted the health-seeking behavior and it is hard to estimate the impacts in terms of morbidity and mortality. While tangible measures are already difficult to account, intangible impacts owing to the pandemic are beyond the scope of the routine data. Surge in severity of diseases, morbidity and mortality of the diseases are some of the indicators that demonstrate the impact of Covid-19 pandemic. In addition, chronic diseases that were on regular follow-up and medication might have been affected by the pandemic as most of the non-serious illnesses were encouraged not to visit the health care centers. Also, people suffering from such chronic diseases including non-acute conditions were scared to visit the health care institutions. Even mild and early cases of Covid-19 felt scared to visit the health center because of the fear and anxiety of being diagnosed as Covid-19-positive patients which might incur stigma and discrimination from family, friends, and the neighbors (Pokharel et al. 2020, Pokharel et al. 2021, Shrestha et al. 2021). Although over the weeks and months, stigma and discrimination against the disease started to falter because majority of the population caught the disease, stigma continued to affect population covertly.

The economic impact from Covid-19 has not been adequately discussed. It is harder to quantify the impact when the parameters that define impact are not so well known. Based on the reports from World Bank, it is estimated that the Covid-19 pandemic is projected to drop the GDP growth, one of the important indicators of healthy economy, by almost 4.5% (~US$4 trillion) (United Nations Development Program 2020). Economic disruption due to to Covid-19 is pervasive and continues to ravage the developing countries' economy that are precariously dependent on everyday businesses. Majority of population in developing countries such as Nepal survive on wages, and daily businesses. Remittance and tourism are the two largest sources of revenue in Nepal which is estimated to have shrunk by 60% and 15 to 20% respectively in 2020. A significant drop in industrial and tourism activities caused three in five employees losing their job in Nepal (United Nations Development Program 2020). A day wasted without work is a day deprived of food. In such settings where population forges food affordability through daily wages or business, impact of Covid-19 itself or the public health measures such as months of lockdowns can have devastating consequences. Food scarcity, further poverty and scores of malnutrition were cautioned by scientists and were reported globally (Singh et al. 2020, Singh et al. 2021).

One of the most heavily affected sectors due to Covid-19 was tourism, transportation, restaurants, movies, and entertainment. Although these sectors apparently do not seem to affect the population health directly, huge proportion of population who were making their livings from the jobs related to these sectors were devastated. As a result, they suffered from irreparable economic loss which impacted on their affordability to routine health care. Additionally, the economic decline has caused mental health issues, which are likely to remain even after the pandemic is brought under control. Apart from these visible economic impacts, there are several hidden economic losses which are hard to estimate and simply might manifest in country's economic indicators. The economic impacts from Covid-19 can more prominently manifest in ongoing infrastructure development.

Development-related works are often underprioritized during such pandemic. The under prioritization can have negative ramifications such as the disruption of the development, freezing of budget and plans, and corruption. Nepal was recovering from the earthquakes of 2015 and rebuilding of Nepal was one of the most discussed topics until the Covid-19 pandemic after which the post-quake rebuilding received much less traction (Adhikari et al. 2016, Mishra and Adhikari 2019, Adhikari, Bhandari et al. 2020, Adhikari, Ozaki et al. 2020). Nearly 7% of houses (out of about 800,000 houses) and 17% of educational institutions (out of some 7,500 educational institutions) remain to be reconstructed even five years after earthquakes. Restoration of heritage sites was also impacted. Apart from the earthquake-related rebuilding, regular development projects have also been halted due to the Covid-19 pandemic. Although some of these projects might have been affected by Covid-19 and the public health measures taken to control the pandemic, many others have been simply put on hold citing the pandemic situation. In fact, projects could have been continued in a controlled fashion. Covid-19 might have offered a space for complacency to pause, delay and invest with a languid effort for the developmental projects.

Learning from the Past and Moving Forward

Nepal's post-pandemic plans for revitalizing social, economic and health sectors relies heavily on its ability to vaccinate, carryout testing and tracing of Covid-19 infections (Stuart et al. 2021). The documented strains of Covid-19 might continue to evolve; therefore, countries like Nepal have no choice but to roll out vaccination that covers the entire population rapidly. Nearly 40% of the population has been vaccinated with at least one dose of Covid-19 vaccines (Covishield, Covaxin, and AstraZeneca) in Nepal thus far. Those waiting to be vaccinated are children and young adults. Given relatively young median age (24.6 years), the young population (aged <40 years) represents nearly 73% of the population, and those aged <20 years represent nearly 40% of the population. They represent the population with higher mobility. Therefore, children and younger adults could still be the driving factor in Covid-19 transmission unless adequately vaccinated.

Nepal has not been able to secure enough vaccines for the entire population, neither through donations nor through purchase (Rankin et al. 2021). The neighboring country Bhutan with a smaller population, has administered nearly three times doses (per 100 people) compared to Nepal (CNN 2021). This is despite the promises made by the government in the past. The political development in the past two years has been increasingly chaotic, with changes in the government resulting in political instability. Multiple procurement processes for testing kits and vaccines have been scarred with corruption charges. At the same time, Nepal's diplomatic efforts to secure vaccine stocks were languishing during the heat of the pandemic. Moreover, vaccine diplomacy was a new experience for developing countries like Nepal. Many vaccine-producing countries were in diplomatic wrangles themselves, casting doubts on their credibility to secure vaccine supplies for poorer countries without any naked self-interest.

Globally, there is no consensus for providing economic and political leeway in producing vaccines locally at a cost that all the countries can always afford. Considering the waning effect of Covid-19 vaccines, multiple vaccination schedules will be required to break the virus transmission cycle reducing infections and deaths. Vaccination and its impacts are essentially dependent on the vaccination coverage which is largely shaped by the public confidence in science, vaccine and efforts to counteract the vaccine hesitancy (Adhikari and Cheah 2021). In addition to promoting the vaccine confidence, it is essential to promote the vaccine production that can meet the global demand. Suspension or removal of patents on Covid-19 vaccines could help decentralize vaccine production, giving a hope for vaccinating the world against Covid-19 (Maxmen 2021, Rankin et al. 2021).

Conclusion

Nepal surmounted a major blow from the 2015 earthquakes by reviving its economy and social sectors until the country was hit by a wave of Covid-19 infections in 2020. Nearly two years into the pandemic, the predicament of poverty, poor governance and widespread corruption has grown out-of-proportion, leaving the country in a dire situation. The country needs to form a sound health and economic recovery plan, one that prioritizes vaccination, contact tracing, and working towards revitalizing the economy. There are important lessons from the Covid-19 pandemic, and like previous disasters, should inform should inform the approaches and strategies for Nepal's health system. Nepal needs to transform its health system response, specifically from reactive to proactive approaches that includes investing and rolling out preparedness efforts for future pandemics. Although proactive and preparatory measures require time, resources and might seem expensive at the outset, in the long run, outcomes are far more economic, effective, and productive.

Acknowledgments

We thank our colleagues, Mukesh Adhikari (University of North Carolina, USA) and Binita Adhikari (Johns Hopkins University, USA), for providing valuable feedback and suggestions.

References

Adhikari, B., P.M. Bhandari, D. Neupane, and S.R. Mishra (2020). "A Retrospective Analysis of Mortality From 2015 Gorkha Earthquakes of Nepal: Evidence and Future Recommendations." *Disaster Med Public Health Prep*: 1–7.

Adhikari, B. and P.Y. Cheah (2021). "Vaccine hesitancy in the COVID-19 era." *Lancet Infect Dis.*, 21(8): 1086.

Adhikari, B. and S.R. Mishra (2016). "Urgent need for reform in Nepal's medical education." *Lancet*, 388(10061): 2739–2740.

Adhikari, B., S.R. Mishra, S. Babu Marahatta, N. Kaehler, K. Paudel, J. Adhikari, and S. Raut (2017). "Earthquakes, Fuel Crisis, Power Outages, and Health Care in Nepal: Implications for the Future." *Disaster Med Public Health Prep.*, 11(5): 625–632.

Adhikari, B., S.R. Mishra and S. Raut (2016). "Rebuilding Earthquake Struck Nepal through Community Engagement." *Front Public Health*, 4: 121.

Adhikari, B., A. Ozaki, S.B. Marahatta, K.R. Rijal, and S.R. Mishra (2020). "Earthquake rebuilding and response to COVID-19 in Nepal, a country nestled in multiple crises." *Journal of Global Health*, 10(2): 020367.

Adhikari, B. et al. (2019). "Treatment-seeking behaviour for febrile illnesses and its implications for malaria control and elimination in Savannakhet Province, Lao PDR (Laos): a mixed method study." *BMC Health Serv Res.*, 19(1): 252.

Al Jazeera. (2021). "How the Delta variant changed the course of the COVID-19 pandemic." Available at https://bit.ly/3xZgNHC. Accessed August 19, 2021.

Amaratunga, D., N. Fernando, R. Haigh, and N. Jayasinghe (2020). "The COVID-19 outbreak in Sri Lanka: A synoptic analysis focusing on trends, impacts, risks and science-policy interaction processes." *Prog Disaster Sci.*, 8: 100133.

Ashish, K.C. et al. (2020). "Effect of the COVID-19 pandemic response on intra-partum care, stillbirth, and neonatal mortality outcomes in Nepal: a prospective observational study." *Lancet Global Health*, 8(10): e1273–e1281.

Ashworth, H.C., T.L. Roux, and C.J.J.I.h. Buggy (2019). "Healthcare accessibility in the rural plains (terai) of Nepal: physical factors and associated attitudes of the local population." 11(6): 528–535.

Awasthi, K.R., K. Adefemi, and M. Tamrakar (2015). "HIV/AIDS: A Persistent Health Issue for Women and Children in Mid and Far Western Nepal." *Kathmandu Univ Med Journal*, 13(49): 88–93.

Bansh Jha, H. (2013). "Nepal's border relations with India and China." *Eurasia Border Review*, 4(1): 63–75.

Bastola, A. et al. (2020). "The first 2019 novel coronavirus case in Nepal." *Lancet Infect Dis.*, 20(3): 279–280.

CNN. (2021). "Tracking Covid-19 vaccinations worldwide." Retrieved September 14, 2021.

Conversation, T. (2020). "What developing countries can teach rich countries about how to respond to a pandemic." Available at https://bit.ly/3ggFhpG. Accessed August 19, 2021.

DW. (2021). "Nepal's delicate balancing act between China and India." Available online at https://bit.ly/3AX3rxe. Accessed August 19, 2021.

El Bcheraoui, C., H. Weishaar, F. Pozo-Martin, and J. Hanefeld (2020). "Assessing COVID-19 through the lens of health systems' preparedness: time for a change." *Global Health*, 16(1): 112.

European Commission. (2020). "Q&A: Coronavirus has shown the need for a global health system – but revealed its weaknesses too." Available at https://bit.ly/3z5MC2S. Accessed August 19, 2021.

Etienne, C. F. et al. (2020). "COVID-19: transformative actions for more equitable, resilient, sustainable societies and health systems in the Americas." *BMJ Global Health*, 5(8).

Ghimire, U., N. Shrestha, B. Adhikari, S. Mehata, Y. Pokharel, and S. R. Mishra (2020). "Health system's readiness to provide cardiovascular, diabetes and chronic respiratory disease related services in Nepal: analysis using 2015 health facility survey." *BMC Public Health*, 20(1): 1163.

Marahatta, S.B. et al. (2020). "Barriers in the access, diagnosis and treatment completion for tuberculosis patients in central and western Nepal: A qualitative study among patients, community members and health care workers." *PLoS One*, 15(1): e0227293.

Maxmen, A.J.N. (2021). "In shock move, US backs waiving patents on COVID vaccines." *Nature*, May 6, 2021. Retrieved August 19, 2021, from www.nature.com/articles/d41586-021-01224-3.

Ministry of Health and Population, Nepal. (2021). "COVID-19 dashboard." Retrieved September 14, 2021, from https://covid19.mohp.gov.np.

Ministry of Health and Population, Nepal. (2020). "Health Sector Emergency Response Plan COVID-19 Pandemic." Retrieved September 12, 2021, from www.who.int/docs/default-source/nepal-documents/novel-coronavirus/health-sector-emergency-response-plan-covid-19-endorsed-may-2020.pdf?sfvrsn=ef831f44_2.

Ministry of Health and Population, Nepal. (2021). "Responding to COVID-19." Available at https://bit.ly/2W5ptPh. Accessed August 19, 2021.

Mishra, S.R. and B. Adhikari (2019). "Planetary health in Nepal's post-earthquake rebuilding agenda: progress and future directions." *Lancet Planet Health*, 3(2): e55–e56.

Mishra, S.R., P. Khanal, D.K. Karki, P. Kallestrup, and U. Enemark (2015). "National health insurance policy in Nepal: challenges for implementation." *Global Health Action*, 8: 28763.

Nepal, B. (2007). "Population mobility and spread of HIV across the Indo-Nepal border." *Journal Health Popul Nutr.*, 25(3): 267–277.

Nepali Times. (2020). "Meanwhile, a measles outbreak in Nepal." Available at www. nepalitimes.com/here-now/meanwhile-a-measles-outbreak-in-nepal. Accessed August 19, 2021.

The New York Times. (2020). "The U.S. and U.K. Were the Two Best Prepared Nations to Tackle a Pandemic—What Went Wrong?" Available online at https:// bit.ly/3dqRGEM. Accessed October 14, 2020.

Pai, M. (2020). "Covidization of research: what are the risks?" *Nat. Med.*, 26(8): 1159.

Pokharel, S., S. Raut, K.R. Rijal, and B. Adhikari (2020). "Coronavirus Disease 2019 Pandemic - Public Health Preparedness in Nepal and One Health Approach." *Disaster Med Public Health Prep*, 15(5), e1-e2..

Poudel, K.C., M. Jimba, J. Okumura, A.B. Joshi and S. Wakai (2004). "Migrants' risky sexual behaviours in India and at home in far western Nepal." *Trop. Med. Int. Health*, 9(8): 897–903.

Rankin, K., D. Citrin, G. Murton, and S. Craig. (2021). "With COVID-19 cases surging, Nepal asks global community for urgent vaccine help." Retrieved September 15, 2021, from https://theconversation.com/with-covid-19-cases-surging-nepal-a sks-global-community-for-urgent-vaccine-help-161333.

Rayamajhee, B. et al. (2021). "How Well the Government of Nepal Is Responding to COVID-19? An Experience From a Resource-Limited Country to Confront Unprecedented Pandemic." *Front Public Health*, 9: 597808.

Rijal, K. R. et al. (2021). "Epidemiology of dengue virus infections in Nepal, 2006–2019." *Infect Dis. Poverty*, 10(1): 52.

Rijal, K. R. et al. (2018). "Epidemiology of Plasmodium vivax Malaria Infection in Nepal." *Am. J. Trop. Med. Hyg.*, 99(3): 680–687.

Sarkar, A., G. Liu, Y. Jin, Z. Xie, and Z.J. Zheng (2020). "Public health preparedness and responses to the coronavirus disease 2019 (COVID-19) pandemic in South Asia: a situation and policy analysis." *Glob Health J.*, 4(4): 121–132.

Sharma, K., A. Banstola, and R.R. Parajuli (2021). "Assessment of COVID-19 Pandemic in Nepal: A Lockdown Scenario Analysis." *Front. Public Health*, 9: 599280.

Shrestha, N. et al. (2021). "Health system preparedness for COVID-19 and its impacts on frontline health care workers in Nepal: a qualitative study among frontline healthcare workers and policymakers." *Disaster Med. Public Health Prep*, 1-9. doi:10.1017/dmp.2021.204.

Singh, D.R., D.R. Sunuwar, B. Adhikari, S. Szabo, and S.S. Padmadas (2020). "The perils of COVID-19 in Nepal: Implications for population health and nutritional status." *J. Glob Health*, 10(1): 010378.

Singh, D.R. et al. (2021). "Impact of COVID-19 on health services utilization in Province-2 of Nepal: a qualitative study among community members and stakeholders." *BMC Health Serv. Res.*, 21(1): 174.

Singh, D.R. et al. (2021). "Food insecurity during COVID-19 pandemic: A genuine concern for people from disadvantaged community and low-income families in Province 2 of Nepal." *PLoS One*, 16(7): e0254954.

Singh, R.P. (2010). "Geo-political position of Nepal and its Impact on Indian Security." *The Indian Journal of Political Science*: 71(4):1281–1292.

Smith, J.L. et al. (2019). "Designing malaria surveillance strategies for mobile and migrant populations in Nepal: a mixed-methods study." *Malaria Journal*, 18(1): 158.

Stuart, R.M. et al. (2021). "Role of masks, testing and contact tracing in preventing COVID-19 resurgences: a case study from New South Wales, Australia." 11(4): e045941.

Tamang, B., P.K. Poudel, S.J. Karki, and R.J.R. Gautam (2020). "A mandatory bonding service program and its effects on the perspectives of young doctors in Nepal." *Rural and Remote Health*, 20(1): 5457–5457.

Udaya Badahur, B.C. et al. (2021). "Anxiety and depression among people living in quarantine centers during COVID-19 pandemic: A mixed method study from western Nepal." *PLoS One*, 16(7): e0254126.

UNICEF. (2020). "More than 117 million children at risk of missing out on measles vaccines, as COVID-19 surges." Statement by the Measles & Rubella Initiative comprising of American Red Cross, US CDC, UNICEF, United Nations Foundation and WHO. Available at www.unicef.org/press-releases/more-117-million-children-risk-missing-out-measles-vaccines-covid-19-surges.

UNICEF. (2021). "No-one is safe until everyone is safe – why we need a global response to COVID-19." Available at https://uni.cf/3z1nHND. Accessed August 19, 2021.

United Nations. (2020). "COVID-19 Exposing Inequalities, Cost of Weak Health, Social Protection Systems, Deputy Secretary-General Tells New York City Webinar Series." Available at https://bit.ly/3jWDe9X. Accessed October 14, 2020.

United Nations Development Program. (2020). "Three in five employees lost their jobs due to COVID-19 in Nepal." Retrieved September 21, 2021 from www.np.undp.org/content/nepal/en/home/presscenter/articles/2020/Three-in-Five-employees-lost-their-jobs-due-to-COVID19-in-Nepal.html.

Vaidya, N.K. and J. Wu (2011). "HIV epidemic in Far-Western Nepal: effect of seasonal labor migration to India." *BMC Public Health*, 11: 310.

The Wall Street Journal. (2021). "Which Countries Have Responded Best to Covid-19?" Available at https://on.wsj.com/2XAjmDf. Accessed August 19, 2021.

World Health Organisation. (2021). "COVID-19 shows why united action is needed for more robust international health architecture." Available at https://bit.ly/37VNwmi. Accessed August 19, 2021.

7 Bangladesh in the Midst of Vaccine Diplomacy

Ali Riaz

Introduction

Bangladesh, like many other countries, experienced adverse economic, social and public health effects of the Covid-19 pandemic; however, since mid-2020, it became a site of contestation between India and China's 'vaccine diplomacy,' that is the use of the Covid-19 vaccine as a tool to enhance their influence over Bangladesh. Both countries offered to provide priority access to the vaccines produced in their respective countries even before the vaccines were approved and manufactured, to ensure that Bangladesh not become dependent on the other country. This chapter examines how the contestation between these two countries played out and locates the rivalry within the larger context of geo-politics of the relationship between Bangladesh and India, and Bangladesh and China.

The Pandemic and its Impact

Bangladesh's first cases of Covid-19 infection were identified in March 2020 (Paul 2020a). The government, like in many other countries was unprepared, although it had the benefit of a three month lag since the global pandemic started. It also repeatedly claimed that it had made all possible preparations to deal with the pandemic. However, the public health system failed to cope with the number of infections; hospitals were woefully ill-equipped to provide care to regular patients as well as those who were infected with Covid-19. Intensive care unit (ICU) beds proved to be scarce (Islam et al. 2020; Al-Zaman 2020). Also, the pace of testing was slow (Cousins 2020). Finally, there was an absence of a coordinated strategy on the part of the government to deal with this public health crisis and its economic fallout. The government's response was a half-hearted lockdown in the form of 'general holiday' in late March.

The economy saw a sudden slump, causing hardship to the middle class and the poorer segments of society. Western buyers of readymade garments (RMG) cancelled orders as the pandemic shut down the economies in Europe and North America. As earnings from the RMG is one of the key pillars of the Bangladeshi economy, these cancellations caused severe loss to

DOI: 10.4324/9781003248149-7

the industry and impacted the workers' jobs and livelihoods. There was a sudden in-migration of laborers from the Gulf. According to government sources, the country lost $1.7bn between March 2020 and June 2021 (*Dhaka Tribune* 2021a).

The Covid-19 pandemic impacted both formal and informal sectors of the economy and resulted in a serious setback to economic growth. The informal sector was the worst hit because millions of workers are involved in it and it constitutes the backbone of the Bangladeshi economy. Hossain (2021) suggests that Covid-19 has pushed 16.5 million people to poverty. These include people who have manual jobs and depends on daily wages, including rickshaw-pullers, transport workers, day laborers, street-vendors, hawkers, construction laborer and the employees of hotel, motel and restaurants. Overall, economists and various organizations have said that it has thrown about 50 million people into poverty in Bangladesh (Uttom 2020). A leading thinktank said overall poverty has risen by 10 percent and could return to a rate of 40 percent, which was the case 15 years ago. In the face of the pandemic, while businesses remained open, the government decided to keep educational institutions closed until September 2021.

Amidst this dire economic backdrop the incumbent Bangladesh Awami League government used the pandemic conditions to silence its critics and clamp down on dissent. The government and the supporters of the ruling party have used the draconian Digital Security Act 2018 as a weapon of persecution (Islam 2021, Riaz 2021).

At the early stages of the Covid-19 outbreak in 2020, the government was far more focused on celebrating the centenary of Sheikh Mujibur Rahman, the founder President of the country and the father of the current Prime Minister Sheikh Hasina. In the subsequent months, with low numbers of recorded deaths, particularly compared to its neighbor India at that time, the incumbent government became complacent, and citizens were negligent about wearing masks and social distancing. Also, the high population density of the country made it difficult to strictly adhere to social distancing norms. Besides, the government's stimulus plans were skewed towards the large businesses and left the small and medium enterprises as well as the poor to fend for themselves (Riaz 2020a, Riaz 2020b). Many were forced to work and defy government restrictions.

In mid-2020, particularly in June, Bangladesh faced a spike in recorded infections as they reached more than 3,500 per day. The spike subsided in subsequent months and contributed to the mistaken impression that the worst was over. By September 2020 there was growing fear that the downward trend of infection was illusory, and the country would face a second wave. Indeed, Prime Minister Sheikh Hasina repeatedly warned of an imminent second wave (*The Daily Star* 2020a), but measures to deal with the inevitable surge were sorely lacking, once again.

In March 2021 the government went ahead with the celebration of the Golden Jubilee of the country and the centenary of Sheikh Mujibur Rahman despite the upward trend of the infections and deaths. Amidst the second wave the government held events with foreign dignitaries including Indian Prime Minister Narendra Modi. Although these events were attended by a small number of guests and audience, for weeks the attention of the government was shifted to these events. Mr. Modi was scheduled to visit the country in 2020 to mark the centenary celebration of Sheikh Mujibur Rahman. The visit was cancelled at that time, owing to the pandemic and protests against his visit (Riaz 2020c). Modi's visit in 2021 took place but was marred by violence leading to at least 14 deaths (Ethirajan, 2021; Amnesty International 2021).

The pandemic situation worsened again in mid-2021; the country faced the third wave with a record number of infections and deaths as the Delta variant spread through the country. Despite warnings of the experts no preventive measures were taken and the country's health care system was overwhelmed (Ahasan and Ravelo 2021). The lack of ICU beds and oxygen supplies caused much suffering and led to the deaths of scores of patients. According to official statistics, by late July 2021 the number of cumulative confirmed cases reached 1.39 million and deaths surpassed 20,000. These official counts underreported deaths and infections, owing to limited testing, the non-inclusion of those who died or remained at home, and the failure to include those who died with Covid-19 symptoms but were not tested before death or recovery.

Search for the Vaccine: India Takes Center Stage

As the efforts to develop vaccines in England by Oxford University with AstraZeneca received a boost and the United States embarked into Operation Warp Speed with Moderna and Pfizer working towards developing the vaccine in March 2020, it became evident that if a vaccine was developed, access to it for the countries with little resources would become a challenge. Discussions and in some measure, concerns, were expressed in Bangladesh as to how the country could ensure access to the vaccine. There were few efforts on the part of the government to ensure access to the vaccine. The low number of infections, an unwillingness to highlight the potential severity of the pandemic and the focus on the celebration of Mujib centennial seem to have precluded the government from taking proactive measures.

The emergence of the global platform COVAX—the Covid-19 Vaccines Global Access Project, which is a global initiative to ensure equitable access to Covid-19 vaccines—in April 2020 was viewed by the Bangladesh's government as the only way to get the vaccine despite calls for contacting the vaccine developers such as AstraZeneca to find ways to procure the vaccines.

In April 2020 the Serum Institute of India (SII), the world's largest vaccine maker, announced its partnership with Oxford University for the production of Covid-19 vaccine. Many in Bangladesh, who were following the development closely viewed this as a positive development hoping that India will share the vaccine with Bangladesh. It is worth noting that the SII was one of the seven global institutions manufacturing the vaccine.

It is against these developments that China offered Bangladesh to conduct its Trial-3 phase of the vaccine CoronaVac, developed by the government firm, Sinovac. On June 21 China invited Bangladesh to receive priority access to a Covid-19 vaccine, once it was developed. On 26 June the Chinese government announced that they might perform second-phase clinical trials of the vaccine in Bangladesh. In July 2020 the Bangladesh Medical Research Council approved Sinovac Biotech to begin a third-phase trial at the International Centre for Diarrheal Disease Research, Bangladesh (Reuters 2020a). The negotiations between the two countries began in July 2020 about conducting the trials from August. However, there was speculation suggesting that India had expressed its displeasure about the cooperation between Bangladesh and China and tried to slow down the process of approval. On August 17, 2020 Indian Foreign Secretary Harsh Vardhan Shringla made a previously unannounced two-day trip to Dhaka—the first since the pandemic began and travel restrictions were imposed. It was reported that "sharing the potential Covid-19 vaccine with Bangladesh is just one of the many promises that had been conveyed by Modi to Sheikh Hasina through Shringla" (Mazumdar 2020).

While China was offering Bangladesh 'priority access' to the vaccine, Bangladesh continued to drag its feet after its initial enthusiasm. It was noted in the Bangladeshi press that "While countries around the world are in hot pursuit of a Covid-19 vaccine, with several currently in the final phase of clinical trials, Bangladesh remains far behind in the race as no desperate effort is visible from the government, experts observed. They said the government has made little progress so far in obtaining the much-sought-after vaccine, as it only submitted an expression of interest as a member of the Global Alliance for Vaccines and Immunisations (GAVI)" (Sujon, 2020).

In India, from May 2020 the SII proceeded with the production of the Astra Zeneca vaccine while waiting for the results of the phase III trial and approval of the country's drug controller (Mint 2021). In late August, a Bangladeshi pharmaceutical company named Beximco reached an investment deal with the SII (Paul 2020b)). The deal, signed on August 28, stipulated 'that Bangladesh is among the first countries to receive an agreed quantity of this vaccine from SII on a priority basis, a BPL statement said... The investment will be treated as an advance for the vaccine' (India TV 2020). Beximco was founded and is led by two brothers, Salman Rahman and Sohail Rahman. Salman Rahman is the Private Sector Industry and Investment Adviser to Prime Minister Sheikh Hasina.

In October 2020 Bangladesh pulled out of the agreement with China regarding the trial, citing differences on cost sharing (DD News 2020). Chinese sources claimed that the delay had compelled them to request cost-sharing, as the original plan to conduct the trial in August was deferred. *The Global Times* reported:

As of October (2020), Sinovac had kicked off clinical trials in some other countries, such as Brazil and Turkey, and could not find external financial support for the clinical trials in Bangladesh, so the company had to negotiate with the Bangladeshi government about sharing the cost to launch the clinical trials. The company had promised to provide free vaccines to Bangladesh for compensation but was refused, according to what *The Global Times* has learned.

(Shumei 2020)

Indian efforts to ensure that Bangladesh received the vaccine exclusively from India came to fruition when a tripartite memorandum of understanding (MOU) was signed between the SII, the Beximco, and the Bangladesh government on November 5 (The Daily Star 2020b). Subsequently, a contract was signed on 13 December 2020. The agreement stipulated that SII would provide 30 million doses of vaccine at the rate of $4, which Beximco would sell to the Bangladesh government for $5. The Bangladesh government immediately paid $153.3 million to the SII (Islam and Sharma 2021). The contract further stipulated that the vaccine would begin to be exported within a month of the approval of the vaccine for use by Bangladesh authorities and would be completed within six months. The contract had no liability clause, thus "if any party, indirectly or due to any special circumstances, face damages, no one will be held liable" (Moral 2021). Although it has not been explicitly expressed, with the signing of the contract Bangladesh became exclusively dependent on SII for the vaccine, except for the vaccines to be received from COVAX. Interestingly, one of the justifications provided by the Bangladesh government for its decision to pull out of the SinoVac trial in August was that it did not want to exclusively rely on a single source of vaccine (DD News 2020).

The Contestation Beyond the Vaccine

The signing of the agreement between these two countries in November was a diplomatic victory for India on two fronts, in terms of halting an apparent slide in relationship with Bangladesh and a pushback to the potential vaccine diplomacy victory of China. In January 2021 India launched the 'Vaccine Maitri' (Vaccine Friendship)—a program that provided vaccines as a humanitarian gesture and on a commercial basis to a number of countries, including Bangladesh.

The relationship between India and Bangladesh has been very close since the Bangladesh Awami League under Sheikh Hasina came into power in 2009. It has been often described as 'special' and 'a Golden era'. The close relationship is due primarily to India's unqualified support to the AL despite its gradual slide to authoritarianism. Yet, in early 2018 some discomfort among Indian policymakers about Bangladesh's growing relationship with China became palpable. In February 2018, Sheikh Hasina had to publicly reassure India that it has nothing to worry about the Bangladeshi-Chinese relationship (The Hindu 2018a). In May 2018, after returning from an official trip to India, Hasina said that India will "remember forever what we have done for them" (Bangla Tribune 2018).

India received unprecedented cooperation from the Hasina regime in rooting out the Northeast Indian insurgents based in Bangladesh during her 2009–14 term. Besides, since her victory in a controversial election in 2014, which was boycotted by all opposition parties, Bangladesh has assiduously met India's demands of providing free transit to Indian goods, allowing the use of Bangladesh's ports, the setting up coastal surveillance system radar, permitting the withdrawal of water from the Feni River and signed a defence cooperation MOU. Bangladesh has taken into consideration the Indian reservations about Chinese involvement in the development of a deep seaport and shelved the project altogether and opted for Japanese investment for a port nearby (Chaudhury 2020).

India's continued support for the Hasina government during the 2018 election which was described by the international press as 'farcical' (The New York Times 2019) and 'transparently fraudulent' (The Economist 2019) helped her weather international criticisms. However, according to Indian press, Hasina was not accorded a proper reception when she visited India twice in 2019 (Roy 2019). According to Indian press, Hasina was received at the airport by a state minister when she visited New Delhi in October 2019, and during her visit to Kolkata in November no central minister or officials came to receive her. These lapses in combination with India's continued disregard for the legitimate concerns of Bangladesh, intensified the prevailing sense of an unequal relationship. Bangladeshis' concerns include water sharing agreement of Teesta River, a reduction of killings on the border by the Indian Border Security Forces of the Bangladeshi citizens alleged to be trying to cross the border and engaged in illicit trade (Kamaruzzaman 2021a), a decrease in the trade imbalance, and the 'Big Brother'-like posturing of India, that is not treating Bangladesh as an equal partner (Riaz 2019a). These issues have contributed to the perception that Bangladesh has conceded more than what it received from India (Kabir 2015, 38). India's siding with the Myanmar government despite the genocide against the Bengali-speaking Rohingya minority has raised questions about the extent of support of India to Bangladesh.

Repeated demeaning comments about Bangladesh by India's Bharatiya Janata Party (BJP) leaders, describing them as 'termites' (The Hindu 2018b; Al Jazeera 2018), and the comment of the Indian Army Chief that Bangladesh was being used as proxy for Pakistan Against India (Scroll.in 2018) were not well-received in Bangladeshis and adversely impacted the image of Indian leaders in Bangladesh. The National Register of Citizenship (NRC) in Assam in August 2019, and the adoption of the Citizenship Amendment Act (CAA) in December 2019 contributed further to tensions in the relationship. The NRC, a database of the citizens of India, was updated in Assam which created serious controversy. The list has made 1.9 million people stateless as they have been left out of the list. Updating the list, originally created in

1951, was demanded by the BJP. It was alleged that it was intended to exclude Muslims in Assam from the list and push them back to Bangladesh (Riaz 2019b). The CAA provides a route to citizenship to members of six religious minority communities from Pakistan, Bangladesh, and Afghanistan—but not for Muslims. As such the law is viewed as discriminatory. Bangladesh government's unease with these measures was evident in the cancellation of visits of Bangladeshi ministers to India (The Indian Express 2019). Although Sheikh Hasina was reportedly satisfied with the assurances from India that Bangladesh has nothing to worry about the NRC, she questioned the necessity of the CAA (The Daily Star 2020c).

By the beginning of 2020 there were ruminations among Indian analysts and the media that the relationship between these two countries warranted New Delhi's special attention as some cracks were becoming visible. A *Hindustan Times* editorial on January 14 noted, "Bangladeshi leaders have expressed their annoyance at how Dhaka has been characterised in Indian discourse and the implications of the [CAA] legislation". The editorial further noted that, "Ms Hasina, [...] has been facing growing criticism in recent months for not getting India to agree to some of Bangladesh's outstanding issues" (Hindustan Times 2020).

Popular perception about India's negative attitude towards Bangladesh became an issue of public discourse and outrage became widespread in social media in June 2021 after a Kolkata based Indian newspaper, the *Anandabazar Patrika* used a derogatory term to describe the Chinese offer of tariff exemptions to 97% of Bangladeshi products (Dhaka Tribune 2020). The report suggested that China was offering 'charity' to woo Bangladesh. Widespread criticisms forced the newspaper to apologize after the Bangladeshi foreign minister weighed in on the matter.

These events and reactions among Bangladeshis, a growing push from China (described below), and a growing reliance of the Bangladesh government on China for investment in infrastructure development had made India concerned. Thus, as the pandemic raged on and the vaccine was being produced in India, it wanted to use it as a tool to keep Bangladesh within its sphere of influence. Bangladesh's decision to stick to India's offer and rely on India for vaccines clearly marked a diplomatic victory for India; at the least for that moment, it succeeded in keeping China at bay. But increasingly there were questions among Bangladeshis whether the Bangladesh government's decision to rely on a singular source was prudent.

The relationship between Bangladesh and China has been a low-key matter for decades despite China being the largest supplier of weapons to Bangladesh since 1978. Cooperation gradually expanded over the past decades, and trade has increased, albeit with a trade deficit in China's favor. The close relationship accelerated since Sino-Indian maritime rivalry intensified. China has viewed Bangladesh as littoral state of the Indian Ocean Region and Bay of Bengal Region and understands its strategic importance. China considers ports on the Bay of Bengal to have strategic value (Anwar 2021). In 2014

Bangladesh agreed to a Chinese proposal to build a deep seaport at Sonadia (bdnews24 2014), but later moved away, owing to India's concerns.

Despite this disappointment, China began aggressively courting Bangladesh from 2016. Resultantly, Bangladesh joined the Belt and Road Initiative (BRI), bought two submarines, signed 26 memoranda of understanding valued at $24.45 billion during the visit of Chinese President Xi Jinping (The Daily Star 2016). To address the Teesta River water issues, Bangladesh asked China for a loan of nearly $1 billion for a comprehensive management and restoration project on the Teesta River (India Today 2020). During the pandemic, Bangladesh reportedly requested $16 billion from China for 26 projects, including nine new projects that were not listed under the BRI. China, Bangladesh's largest trading partner, has also reduced tariffs for 97 percent of Bangladeshi imported products under its Preferential Tariff Program in June 2020. The relationship is now described as a "strategic partnership for cooperation." (NDTV 2020) From economic and strategic standpoints, China considers Bangladesh as an essential nodal point for its influence in South Asia. As noted by an analyst, 'the Bangladesh-China-India-Myanmar Economic Corridor—one of the six proposed economic corridors of China's BRI—relies on Bangladesh as a central location' (Anwar 2021).

It is against this background that China saw the supply of vaccines as an opportunity to bring Bangladesh deeply into its sphere of influence. The ongoing trial of its vaccine, ahead of other potential vaccines, bolstered its efforts in mid-2020.

The bilateral relationship between Bangladesh and India on the one hand and Bangladesh and China on the other, and the ongoing rivalry between China and India had put Bangladesh in the middle of a tug-of-war, but it was also part of the geopolitical agendas of these countries which made Bangladesh a site of contestation. India's decision to use Covid-19 as a tool, especially in the region, was predicated by its inability to match China's deep pockets. As noted by Chatterjee et al. (2021, 361):

> Lacking the kind of economic resources that China commands, India's efforts to match that influence have been largely ineffective thus far. From the point of view of international diplomacy, one cannot, therefore, blame India to take advantage of her resources and extend her geo-political diplomacy, even if that comes at a time of global health crises. It is undeniable that India's vaccine gifts will serve to polish its global image and earn her goodwill, especially in South Asia where it is often criticized for its 'big brother' behaviour.

The question of India's image in the region is worth underscoring. In addition to the longstanding problem of being perceived as intrusive by its neighbors, in recent years, particularly since BJP came into power, India is viewed negatively by its neighbors (Ganguly 2020). India's domestic developments, particularly the undemocratic behavior of the Modi government through its adoption of the highly discriminatory laws such as CAA, the ruling BJP supporters' attacks on minorities, have contributed to this image. Besides, a significant number of population in Bangladesh, Nepal, and Sri Lanka, feel that India has pursued its own interests at the expense of democracy in their respective countries.

One can hardly ignore the geostrategic considerations of India in selecting the countries for priority access. Wrapped around the 'neighborhood first' policy, the countries which received the first batch of supply of vaccine after India launched the 'Vaccine Maitri' included "Nepal, Bhutan, Bangladesh as well as the Indian Ocean nations of Sri Lanka, Maldives, Mauritius and Seychelles - all important elements in India's geostrategic calculus" (Chandra 2021). Prioritization of the bilateral mode of distribution of vaccines is a clear indication that it is intended to improve relationships and gain influence. *Vaccine Maitri's* global dimension was designed to send a message to the global community that in the emergent new global order, India as a middle power was dependable and responsible actor.

While India's vaccine diplomacy in South Asia was intended to rebuild its relationships, China had two distinct objectives; first, to establish itself as a regional 'friend in need' and second, to offer a product which helps to lessen dependency on the West. It is the latter which became the hallmark of China's efforts since the pandemic began. In the early days it provided Personal Protective Equipment, testing kits and doctors to several countries and invested in research and development to develop a vaccine at the same time other vaccines were in the development stage. Its transnational trials were intended to gain trust about its product. These strategies paid off as, by March 2021, despite concerns about the efficacy, Chinese vaccines swept much of the world (Wu and Gelineau 2021).

The Beginning, the Hiccup, the Disruption, and a Sharp Turn

The signing of the deal with the SII in November 2020 was portrayed by the Bangladesh Government as a success of its diplomacy and the farsightedness of Prime Minister Hasina. It implied that its close relationship with India had paid off at a very difficult time. As India launched the *Vaccine Maitri* in January and Bangladesh was on the list of countries with priority access to the vaccine, cabinet ministers and ruling party leaders described it as a victory in the battle against Covid-19. The prevailing impression was that a steady stream of vaccines from India coupled with future allocations from COVAX would enable the country to confront the pandemic head on.

However, the first hiccup came on January 3, 2021, when Adar Poonawalla, the CEO of the SII told the Associated Press that the company would not be able to sell vaccines on the private market until March or April. He cited the conditions imposed by the Indian authorities in granting emergency authorization (Ghosal 2021). Although such a decision would have affected not only Bangladesh but would have placed COVAX in a difficult spot, reactions in Bangladesh were quite strong. The decision was viewed as another of India's unkept promises (Mukhopadhyay 2021). Nevertheless, the SII later clarified the decision and assured that the company will honor its commitment to the private buyers and to COVAX. On January 21, Bangladesh received two million doses of the SII manufactured CoviShield vaccine as a gift from India, and four days later, five million doses were delivered as the first batch of delivery under the contract.

Based on the vaccines on hand and the promises of steady supply from SII under the contract, Bangladesh launched the inoculation drive on February 5 (Paul 2021). It received the second batch of two million doses on February 22. When Narendra Modi visited Bangladesh on March 26, he gifted another 1.2 million doses. Before another hundred thousand doses were gifted by the Indian Army Chief Mukund Narvane to his counterpart during his visit to Dhaka on April 8, India was facing the devastating second wave of the pandemic. International media reported on March 24 that the government had decided to suspend vaccine exports (The Wall Street Journal 2021; BBC 2021). Thus, although Bangladesh was supposed to receive five million vaccines per month, by early April when India stopped exporting the vaccine the total number received altogether fell to 10.3 million doses and the country faced enormous uncertainty. In April, one government official expressed the fear that Bangladesh could face problems with the second dose of the vaccines as the supplies from India were yet to arrive. Although the health minister later assured that there was no shortage of the vaccine, Bangladesh had to stop its inoculation drive on April 25, 2021.

Empty assurances failed to allay the growing concerns; instead, criticisms of the government for relying on a single source grew louder, the managing director of the Beximco—a ruling party leader—Nazmul Hasan Papon angrily complained, "Serum Institute has no right to halt vaccine supply after Bangladesh paid in advance" (The Daily Star 2021a). It was reported in the press that Bangladesh's repeated efforts to get a clear answer as to when SII would resume exports remained unanswered even as the Bangladeshi Foreign Minister reached out to his Indian counterpart (Kamaruzzaman 2021b).

The Bangladesh government launched a frantic effort for an alternative source in late April and contacted China and Russia. Previously, the Russian requests for approval of its Sputnik V had received a cold shoulder from Bangladesh. In early April, it also offered a co-production deal. Bangladeshi drug regulator approved the Sputnik V and SinoVac for emergency use on 27 and 29 April 2021 respectively (Dhaka Tribune 2021b).

With the arrival of the first batch of 500,000 SinoVac vaccines as a gift on May 12, followed by another 600,000 on June 13, Bangladesh made a sharp turn about the source of vaccines. On June 12 Bangladesh signed a deal with China. The deal was signed after some confusion and misunderstandings about the violation of the Non-Disclosure Agreement. On 27 May after the deal was approved by a Cabinet Committee on Public Purchase a government official divulged the rate of the vaccine which Beijing did not like (Dhaka Tribune 2021c).

In the meantime, Bangladesh appealed to the international community for help and expressed displeasure that the vaccine was being used as 'tool of exploitation' (Dhaka Tribune 2021d). The Bangladeshi Foreign Minister alleged that "they [rich countries] assure us just saying, 'you don't worry,' but nobody gives us vaccines. In some cases, they want to know whether we [Bangladesh] will support them on a particular issue [various elections in global forums]" (Dhaka Tribune 2021d). Bangladesh began to receive Pfizer-BioNTech vaccines through COVAX facilities on May 31, and later the United States began to send Moderna vaccines as a gift (Reuters 2021).

Conclusion: Implications and Trajectories

The cascade of events since Summer of 2020 in the backdrop of an ongoing tussle between India and China to extend their spheres of influence placed Bangladesh in the middle of a tug-of-war using the Covid-19 vaccine. While India, in the first round of vaccine diplomacy, scored against China and kept China at bay, the catastrophic second wave in April 2021 in India, combined with the ill planning of its *Vaccine Maitri*, created the opportunity for China. This was equally true for other countries in the region. India's failure to provide vaccines, especially when Bangladesh was exclusively dependent on it and it did not explore other sources, owing to India's discouragement, will have a serious backlash in the future.

It is important to remember that the Indo-Bangladesh relationship has been far more complex as noted by Bhushan there is "a widening gap between the excellent functional relationship between the two governments and the perception of the people of Bangladesh" (Bhushan 2021). The negative perception is rooted in India's role in the domestic politics of Bangladesh, especially its unqualified support to the incumbent Awami League despite democratic backsliding. In the future, vaccines could help India to demonstrate that it intends to help Bangladesh in its efforts to fight against the pandemic, and push back the growing influence of China, but it will take more than vaccines to change the perception of Bangladeshis of India as a hegemonic and overbearing neighbor with an agenda to dominate the region and influence its domestic politics.

Vaccine diplomacy has not only cemented the relationship between Bangladesh and China, but it has provided additional leverage to the latter. The end of the pandemic is unlikely to diminish its growing influence. China's posture toward Bangladesh, neither before nor during the pandemic, has been benign. China has been playing a long game and made serious headway before the pandemic, thanks to its deep pockets and dazzling investments which helped the ruling Bangladesh Awami League (BAL) justify its undemocratic behavior through performance legitimacy. The Hasina government is engaged in a balancing act and argues that the relationship with China is economic while the relationship with India is political. Whether such a bifurcation is possible remains an open question. Besides, it is also worth considering whether the BAL now feels more ideological affinity to China than India.

China is taking a more assertive posture towards Bangladesh as demonstrated in comments made by the Chinese Ambassador to Bangladesh. On May 10, in a press conference in Dhaka, Ambassador Li Jiming warned that if Bangladesh joins the "small club of four [the Quad], it will substantially damage our bilateral relationship" (The Print 2021). The Quadrilateral Security Dialogue, referred to as the Quad, was initiated in 2017 with the US, Japan, Australia and India as its members. China views it as "a military alliance aimed at countering China's resurgence" and has described it as a "narrow purposed geopolitical group." (*Bangkok Post* 2021) The Bangladeshi Foreign Minister A. K. Momen immediately rebuffed the suggestion that the country had any plans to join the group and asserted its non-aligned foreign policy. In his response Momen said, "We're an independent and sovereign state. We decide our foreign policy" (The Print 2021). United States' Department of State spokesperson reacted saying that the "US has taken note of the comment" (The Daily Star 2021b). Nevertheless, Chinese Foreign Ministry spokesperson later stood by its envoy's characterization of the Quad, although she did not comment on whether China has warned Bangladesh. This comment came on the heels of the Chinese Defense minister Wei Fenghe's plea to the Bangladeshi President Abdul Hamid on April 27 during a meeting to not join the Quad. Wei urged Bangladesh to "take joint efforts against the formation of a military alliance led by the United States for maintaining 'hegemony' in South Asia" (Chowdhury 2021).

China's move to take advantage of the pandemic situation is not only limited to Bangladesh; instead, China has taken the initiative to create an institutional structure involving five South Asian countries, namely Afghanistan, Pakistan, Nepal, Sri Lanka, and Bangladesh. The initiative excludes India. The China-South Asia Emergency Supplies Reserve was launched on July 9, 2021. China also established a center for cooperation on poverty reduction and development. Evidently these efforts will complement China's BRI project.

The contestation between these two countries in the region will continue in coming days as these countries will need the vaccines for millions of people. For example, with more than 160 million people, of which more than 104 million are adults, Bangladesh's required number of vaccines are unlikely to be received from COVAX facilities. With the improvement of India's pandemic situation the SII will be able to supply vaccines to Bangladesh later in the year. However, it will now have to compete with China and Russia. China has already invested in vaccine development and has its own vaccines to share including engaging in coproduction in Bangladesh, while India will not be able to replicate the Chinese strategy. The contestation will not remain limited with the vaccine supply but will involve other spheres.

One of the critical factors for the ongoing contestation between India and China in Bangladesh has been due to the conspicuous absence of the United States in the past decade. Despite the US being the single largest market of Bangladeshi goods in the world and having robust security and anti-terrorism cooperative arrangements with the country, it seems to have little leverage over Bangladesh. Beyond economic and security cooperation, the US has relied on India in pursuing its interests. Considering the changed circumstances—a gradual decline of India's democratic credentials, a lack of trust of India on the part of Bangladesh's citizens, the devastation caused by the pandemic, and its lack of economic prowess to match the assertive moves of China, it might be time for the US to reconsider its approach to Bangladesh. The delivery of vaccines by the United States at a crucial time was a welcome development, from both humanitarian and diplomatic perspectives. The future trajectory of the post-Covid-19 Bangladesh will depend on whether the Biden administration is willing to enhance its engagement with Bangladesh, otherwise a far more intense contestation between China and India, the scale albeit tilting towards the former, along with growing authoritarianism of the incumbent in domestic politics, is the most likely scenario.

References

Al Jazeera. 2018. "BJP chief slammed for calling Bangladeshi migrants "termites."" September 24, 2018, www.aljazeera.com/news/2018/9/24/bjp-chief-slammed-for-ca lling-bangladeshi-migrants-termites. Accessed July 4, 2021.

Ahasan, Nazmul and Jenny Lei Ravelo. 2021. "Bangladesh battles third wave of COVID-19." *Devex*, July 14, 2021. www.devex.com/news/bangladesh-battles-third-wave-of-COVID-19-100340. Accessed July 19, 2021.

Al-Zaman, Md. Sayeed, 2020. "Healthcare Crisis in Bangladesh during the COVID-19 Pandemic." *American Journal of Tropical Medicine*, 103(4): 1357–1359, August 2020, www.ncbi.nlm.nih.gov/pmc/articles/PMC7543838/. Accessed June 30, 2021.

Amnesty International. 2021. "Bangladesh authorities must conduct prompt, thorough, impartial, and independent investigations into the death of protesters and respect people's right to peaceful assembly." April 1, 2021, www.amnesty.org/en/la test/news/2021/04/bangladesh-protests-statement/. Accessed 17 July 2021.

Anwar, Anu. 2021. "Bangladesh at 50: Navigating Strategic Survival." *War on the Rocks*, April 26, 2021. https://warontherocks.com/2021/04/bangladesh-at-50-naviga ting-strategic-survival/ Accessed July 21, 2021.

Bangkok Post. 2021. "Why China is anxious about the Quad." May 24, 2021. www. bangkokpost.com/business/2120627/why-china-is-anxious-about-the-quad Accessed August 21, 2021.

Bangla Tribune. 2018. "India will never forget what we did for them." May 10, 2018, https://en.banglatribune.com/national/news/3763/%E2%80%98India-will-always-rem ember-what-we-did-for-them%E2%80%99. Accessed June 21, 2021.

BBC. 2021. "Coronavirus: India temporarily halts Oxford-AstraZeneca vaccine exports." March 24, 2021. www.bbc.com/news/world-asia-india-56513371. Accessed March 26, 2021.

Bdnews24. 2014. "Sonadia deep-sea port on board." June 8, 2014. https://bdnews24. com/economy/2014/06/08/sonadia-deep-sea-port-on-board. Accessed July 1, 2021.

Bhushan, Bharat. 2021. "Dhaka disconnect: Excellent relations marred by violent protests." *Business Standard*, Match 29, 2021. www.business-standard.com/article/op inion/dhaka-disconnect-excellent-relations-marred-by-violent-protests-121032900101_ 1.html Accessed April 2, 2021.

Chandra, Purabi. 2021. "As "Vaccine Maitri" flops, China steps in." *Deccan Herald*, June 1, 2021. www.deccanherald.com/opinion/in-perspective/as-vaccine-maitri-flop s-china-steps-in-992307.html. Accessed July 2, 2021.

Chatterjee, Niladri, Zaad Mahmood, and Eleanor Marcussen. 2021. "Politics of Vaccine Nationalism in India: Global and Domestic Implications." *Forum for Development Studies*, 48(2): 357–369.

Chaudhury, Dipanjan Roy. 2020. "Bangladesh drops plan to develop a deep-sea port at Sonadia island." *The Economic Times*, October 15, 2020, https://econom ictimes.indiatimes.com/news/international/world-news/bangladesh-drops-plan-to-develo p-a-deep-sea-port-at-sonadia-island/articleshow/78688376.cms?utm_source=contentofin terest&utm_medium=text&utm_campaign=cppst Accessed August 27, 2021.

Chowdhury, Shahidul Islam. 2021. "China seeks Bangladesh support against US-led military alliance in South Asia." *New Age*, April 29, 2021. www.newagebd.net/article/ 136658/china-seeks-support-against-us-led-military-alliance-in-south-asia.   Accessed April 30, 2021.

Cousins, Sophie. 2020. "Bangladesh's COVID-19 testing criticized." *Lancet*, 396, August 29, 2020. www.thelancet.com/journals/lancet/article/PIIS0140-6736(20) 31819-5/fulltext. Accessed September 15, 2020.

DD News. 2020. "Bangladesh not to prioritise Chinese COVID 19 Vaccine trial." August 4, 2020. http://ddnews.gov.in/international/bangladesh-not-prioritise-chinese-COVID-19-vaccine-trial. Accessed April 2, 2021.

Dhaka Tribune. 2020. "97% Bangladeshi products to get duty-free access to China." June 19, 2021. www.dhakatribune.com/business/2020/06/19/5-161-more-bangladeshi-p roducts-to-enjoy-zero-tariff-to-chinese-markets-from-july-1. Accessed May 23, 2021.

Dhaka Tribune. 2021a. "PM: Bangladesh's economy lost $17bn to COVID-19." June 29, 2021. www.dhakatribune.com/business/economy/2021/06/29/pm-budget-imp lementable-will-take-bangladesh-a-step-forward. Accessed June 30, 2021.

Dhaka Tribune. 2021b. "For now, Bangladesh stopping first dose of COVID vaccine from Monday." April 25, 2021. www.dhakatribune.com/bangladesh/2021/04/25/ba ngladesh-to-stop-administering-first-dose-of-vaccine-from-april-26 Accessed August 30, 2021.

Dhaka Tribune. 2021c. "COVID-19: Bangladesh signs deal with China to buy vaccines." June 12, 2021. www.dhakatribune.com/bangladesh/foreign-affairs/2021/06/12/COV ID-19-bangladesh-signs-deal-with-china-to-buy-vaccines. Accessed June 14, 2021.

Dhaka Tribune. 2021d. "FM Moment: COVID vaccine apparently emerged as another tool of exploitation." June 22, 2021.

The Economist. 2019. "Obituary of a democracy: Bangladesh." January 30, 2019. https:// espresso.economist.com/0390aff9c68eeb7b64fbebe21c878de3. Accessed April 2, 2021.

Ethirajan, Anbarasan. 2021. "Why Narendra Modi's visit to Bangladesh led to 12 deaths." *BBC News*, March 31, 2021. www.bbc.com/news/world-asia-56586210. Accessed July 11, 2021.

Ganguly, Sumit. 2020. "India Is Paying the Price for Neglecting its Neighbors." *Foreign Policy*, June 23, 2020. https://foreignpolicy.com/2020/06/23/india-china-south-asia-relations/. Accessed May 15, 2021.

Ghosal, Aniruddha. 2021. "AP Interview: India bars virus vaccine maker from exporting." January 3, 2021. https://apnews.com/article/ap-top-news-global-trade-immunizations-india-coronavirus-pandemic-c0c881c0f07166e8fd494e078171a7cc. Accessed March 5, 2021.

Hindustan Times. 2020. "Reassure Dhaka; bring ties back on track." January 14, 2020. www.hindustantimes.com/editorials/reassure-dhaka-bring-ties-back-on-track/story-PHF6frQSgFdelDm8YPibUJ.html. Accessed July 21, 2021.

Hossain, Mohammad Imran. 2021. "COVID-19 Impacts on Employment and Livelihood of Marginal People in Bangladesh: Lessons Learned and Way Forward," *South Asian Survey*, 28(1): 57–71. March 2021.

India TV. 2020. "Bangladesh's pharma company Beximo announces investment plans with India's SIL." August 30, 2020. www.indiatvnews.com/news/good-news/bangladesh-s-pharma-company-beximo-announces-investment-plans-with-india-s-sil-645913. Accessed May 5, 2021.

Indian Express. 2019. "Bangladesh ministers cancel visit to India." December 13, 2019, https://indianexpress.com/article/india/bangladesh-ministers-cancel-visit-to-india-citizenship-amendment-bill-6164430/. Accessed June 25, 2021.

India Today. 2020. "China to lend Bangladesh almost $1 billion for Teesta River project, reports Bangladeshi media." August 17, 2020. www.indiatoday.in/world/story/china-to-lend-bangladesh-almost-1-billion-for-teesta-river-project-reports-bangladeshi-media-1712284-2020-08-17. Accessed July 5, 2021.

Islam, Arafatul. 2021. "How is Bangladesh's Digital Security Act muzzling free speech?" Deutsche Welle, March 3, 2021. www.dw.com/en/how-is-bangladeshs-digital-security-act-muzzling-free-speech/a-56762799. Accessed April 4, 2021.

Islam, Sufia, Rizwanul Islam, Fouzia Mannan, Sabera Rahman, and Tahiya Islam. 2020. "COVID-19 pandemic: An analysis of the healthcare, social and economic challenges in Bangladesh." *Progress in Disaster*, 8, December 2020; www.sciencedirect.com/science/article/pii/S2590061720300727. Accessed July 16, 2021.

Islam, Syful and Kiran Sharma. 2021. "India COVID spike pushes Bangladesh to tap Sputnik and Sinopharm." Nikkei Asia, May 7, 2021. https://asia.nikkei.com/Spotlight/Coronavirus/India-COVID-spike-pushes-Bangladesh-to-tap-Sputnik-and-Sinopharm. Accessed July 20, 2021.

Kabir, Humayun. 2015. "Changing Relations Between Bangladesh and India; Perception in Bangladesh." in *India and South Asia: Exploring Regional Perceptions*, ed. Yishal Chandra. New Delhi: IDSA and Pentagon Press.

Kamaruzzaman, Md. 2021a. "Unlawful killings' along India border: Bangladeshi families seek justice." Anadolu Agency, February 11, 2021. www.aa.com.tr/en/asia-pacific/unlawful-killings-along-india-border-bangladeshi-families-seek-justice/2141343 Accessed August 25, 2021.

Kamaruzzaman, Md. 2021b. "Bangladesh urges India for immediate release of purchased vaccines." Anadolu Agency, May 19, 2021. www.aa.com.tr/en/asia-pacific/bangladesh-urges-india-for-immediate-release-of-purchased-vaccines/2246573#. Accessed July 20, 2021.

Mazumdar, Jaideep. 2020. "Explained: The Reasons Behind Indian Foreign Secretary's Sudden Visit To Bangladesh This Week." *Swarajya*, August 21, 2020. https://

swarajyamag.com/world/explained-the-reasons-behind-indian-foreign-secretarys-sud den-visit-to-bangladesh-this-week. Accessed April 1, 2021.

mint. 2020. "Serum Institute produced 5,000 doses of Covishield every minute. A look at vaccine journey." January 16, 2021. www.livemint.com/news/india/ 5000-doses-of-covishield-minute-a-look-at-serum-institutes-s-vaccine-journey-11610809058833.html. Accessed July 19, 2021.

Moral, Shishir. 2021. "Serum Vaccine: Contract has non-liability clause." *Prothom Alo English*. May 7, 2021. https://en.prothomalo.com/bangladesh/serum-vaccine-contract-has-non-liability-clause. Accessed June 30, 2021.

Mukhopadhyay, Ankita. 2021. "Why the Bangladesh-India friendship is under pressure." *Deutsche Welle*, February 5, 2021. www.dw.com/en/india-bangladesh-ties/a -56473457. Accessed March 5, 2021.

NDTV. 2020. "Ready To Take China-Bangladesh Strategic Partnership To New Heights: Xi Jinping." October 4, 2020. www.ndtv.com/world-news/ready-to-ta ke-china-bangladesh-strategic-partnership-to-new-heights-xi-jinping-2304919 Acces sed October 29, 2021.

The New York Times. 2019. "Bangladesh's Farcical Vote." January 14, 2019, www. nytimes.com/2019/01/14/opinion/editorials/bangladesh-election-sheikh-hasina.html. Accessed March 23, 2021.

Parvez, Sohel. 2020. "Pandemic doubles extreme poverty." *The Daily Star*, July 19, 2020. www.thedailystar.net/business/news.pandemic-doubles-extreme-poverty-1943653. Acce ssed July 16, 2021.

Paul, Ruma. 2021. "The wait is over": Bangladesh begins COVID-19 vaccinations." Reuters, February 7, 2021. www.reuters.com/business/healthcare-pharmaceuticals/ the-wait-is-over-bangladesh-begins-COVID-19-vaccinations-2021-02-07/. Accessed June 8, 2021.

Paul, Ruma. 2020a. "Bangladesh confirms its first three cases of coronavirus." *Reuters*, March 8, 2020. www.reuters.com/article/us-health-coronavirus-bangladesh/bangla desh-confirms-its-first-three-cases-of-coronavirus-idUSKBN20V0FS. Accessed April 4, 2021.

Paul. Ruma. 2020b. "Bangladesh's Beximco signs COVID-19 vaccine deal with India's Serum Institute." Reuters. August 28, 2020. www.reuters.com/article/us-health-cor onavirus-bangladesh-india/bangladeshs-beximco-signs-COVID-19-vaccine-deal-with-indias-serum-institute-idUSKBN25O1HT Accessed July 10, 2021.

Reuters. 2020a. "Bangladesh to Host Late-Stage Trial of China's Sinovac COVID-19 Vaccine." July 20, 2020. www.reuters.com/article/us-health-coronavirus-bangla desh/bangladesh-to-host-late-stage-trial-of-chinas-sinovac-COVID-19-vaccine-i dUSKCN24L0KO. Accessed April 2, 2021.

Reuters. 2021. "White House says 2.5 million doses of Moderna will begin to ship to Bangladesh Tuesday." June 29, 2021. www.reuters.com/business/healthcare-pharma ceuticals/white-house-says-25-million-doses-moderna-will-begin-ship-bangladesh-tuesda y-2021-06-29. Accessed August 30, 2021.

Riaz, Ali. 2020. "Modi's canceled Bangladesh visit is an opportunity." *New Atlanticist*, March 10, 2020. www.atlanticcouncil.org/blogs/new-atlanticist/modis-canceled-bangla desh-visit-is-an-opportunity. Accessed July 1, 2021.

Riaz, Ali. 2020a. "Bangladesh's COVID-19 stimulus: Leaving the most vulnerable behind." *New Atlanticist*, April 8, 2020. www.atlanticcouncil.org/blogs/new-atlanticist/ bangladeshs-COVID-19-stimulus-leaving-the-most-vulnerable-behind/. Accessed June 10, 2021.

Riaz, Ali. 2020b. "A Tale of Misplaced Priorities." *The Daily Star*, July 12, 2020. www.thedailystar.net/opinion/black-white-grey/news/tale-misplaced-prio rities-1928729. Accessed July 7, 2021.

Riaz, Ali. 2019a. "The Indo-Bangladesh Relationship; "Saath Saath" (Together) or Too Close for Comfort?" *Indian Politics and Policy*, 2(1): 53–75, Spring 2009.

Riaz, Ali. 2019b. "NRC in Assam: What Happened? What's Next?". *The Daily Star*, September 8, 2019. www.thedailystar.net/opinion/black-white-and-grey/news/nrc-a ssam-what-happened-whats-next-1796872. Accessed August 28, 2021.

Riaz, Ali. 2021. "How Bangladesh's Digital Security Act Is Creating a Culture of Fear." Carnegie Endowment for International Peace, December 9, 2021. Retrieved February 2, 2022, from https://carnegieendowment.org/2021/12/09/how-bangla desh-s-digital-security-act-is-creating-culture-of-fear-pub-85951.

Roy, Agni. 2019. "Cold Reception to Ally Hasina: Delhi is on the Dock." (in Bengali) *Anandabazar Patrika*. www.anandabazar.com/india/critics-slam-modi-government-for-not-welcoming-sheikh-hasina-properly-1.1074577. Accessed March 24, 2021.

Scroll.in. 2018. "Army chief says Assam's AIUDF has grown at a faster pace than the BJP." February 22, 2018. https://scroll.in/latest/869584/army-chief-blames-pakista n-china-for-planned-migration-from-bangladesh-into-northeast-india, Accessed July 5, 2021.

Shumei, Leng. 2021. "India meddling behind halt of Sinovac vaccine trials in Bangla desh: source." *Global Times*, January 26, 2021. www.globaltimes.cn/page/202101/ 1214041.shtml. Accessed April 3, 2021.

Sujan, Moudud Ahmmed. 2020. "Bangladesh in Vaccine Race: Way behind." *The Daily Star*, August 26, 2020. www.thedailystar.net/frontpage/news/bangladesh-vacci ne-race-way-behind-1951021. Accessed July 15, 2020.

The Daily Star. 2020a. "*PM again warns of second wave.*" November 19, 2020. www. thedailystar.net/frontpage/news/pm-again-warns-COVID-2nd-wave-1997253. Acces sed July 1, 2021.

The Daily Star. 2020b. "Buying 3cr Vaccine Doses: Govt signs deal with India's SII, Beximco Pharma." November 6, 2020. www.thedailystar.net/frontpage/news/ buying-3cr-vaccine-doses-govt-signs-deal-indias-sii-beximco-pharma-1990077. Acces sed July 1, 2021.

The Daily Star. 2020c. "India's CAA unnecessary, says prime minister."January 20, 2020. www.thedailystar.net/frontpage/india-citizenship-law-unnecessary-1856419/ Accessed June 25, 2021.

The Daily Star. 2021a. "Serum Institute has no right to halt vaccine supply after Ban gladesh paid in advance: Papon."April 24, 2021. www.thedailystar.net/coronavir us-deadly-new-threat/news/serum-institute-has-no-right-halt-vaccine-supply-after-ba ngladesh-paid-advance-papon-2082969. Accessed April 25, 2012.

The Daily Star. 2021b. "US takes note of China envoy's comment on Quad to Ban gladesh."May 12, 2021. www.thedailystar.net/us/news/us-takes-note-china-envoys-comment-quad-bangladesh-2092613. Accessed May 13, 2021.

The Hindu. 2018a. "India has. nothing to worry about China-Bangla ties: Sheikh Hasina."February 21, 2018. www.thehindu.com/news/international/india-has-noth ing-to-worry-about-china-bangla-ties-sheikh-hasina/article22813370.ece.   Accessed July 15, 2021.

The Hindu. 2018b. "Bangladeshi migrants are like termites: Amit Shah."September 22, 2018.   www.thehindu.com/news/national/bangladeshi-migrants-are-like-termites-am it-shah/article25017064.ece. Accessed July 4, 2021.

The Print. 2021. "China warns Bangladesh of "substantial damage" to relations if it joins US-led Quad alliance."May 11, 2021. https://theprint.in/diplomacy/china-warns-bangladesh-of-substantial-damage-to-relations-if-it-joins-us-led-quad-alliance/656403. Accessed May 12, 2021.

Uttom, Stephan. 2021. "COVID-19 to throw millions into poverty in Bangladesh." UCA News. April 16, www.ucanews.com/news/COVID-19-to-throw-millions-into-poverty-in-bangladesh/87737#. Accessed August 28, 2021.

Wall Street Journal. 2021. "India Suspends COVID-19 Vaccine Exports to Focus on Domestic Immunization." www.wsj.com/articles/india-suspends-COVID-19-vaccine-exports-to-focus-on-domestic-immunization-11616690859. Accessed March 23, 2021.

Wu, Huizhong and Kristen Gelineau. 2021. "Chinese vaccines sweep much of the world, despite concerns." Associated Press, March 1, 2021. https://apnews.com/article/china-vaccines-worldwide-0382aefa52c75b834fbaf6d869808f51. Accessed April 2, 2021.

8 Fallout from the Pandemic: the Experience of Indian Diasporas in the Gulf States

Nicolas Blarel

The Experience of Indian Diasporas in the Gulf States

Since March 2020, the massive global outbreak of novel coronavirus (Covid-19) pandemic has disrupted the Gulf economies, as a consequence notably of the dual shock of the long-term collapse of oil prices and the abrupt spread of the pandemic. Oil prices had already drastically dropped over the last decade with the average yearly crude oil price plummeting from around $98 per barrel in 2013 to less than $40 per barrel in 2020. This already had a massive direct income effect on the Gulf Cooperation Council (GCC) countries. The IMF forecasted an average 7.1 percent drop in GCC's GDP in 2020.[1] The Covid-19 pandemic has further exacerbated this difficult situation by affecting both supply and demand, by considerably disrupting the global supply chains and limiting the global demand for oil.

The combination of the sanitary and economic crises severely impacted the living and working conditions of the vast majority of expatriates in the urban Gulf. The Gulf states of Bahrain, Kuwait, Oman, Qatar, United Arab Emirates (UAE), and Saudi Arabia all imposed various restrictive measures to control and prevent the spread of Covid-19 outbreak. Key measures included but were not limited to mass Covid-19 testing, temporary lockdowns and curfews, market closures, significant fines and penalties, public health campaigns in high-risk accommodation spaces, notably labour camps.[2] As Covid-19 cases rose, the GCC states were forced to close their major industries, including construction, retail, manufacturing, and other service-based sectors which inevitably led to the massive unemployment for all foreign workers.

As a result, labour- sending states—specifically India, Pakistan, Sri Lanka, Nepal, the Philippines, and Bangladesh—have immediately facilitated the repatriation of their nationals. However, the vast supply of foreign workers has remained in the Gulf, owing to perceived weak economic prospects and opportunities in their home states, as well as the expectations that Gulf economies would quickly recover from the economic recession. Given the financial instability and the prolonged spread of Covid-19, the GCC private

DOI: 10.4324/9781003248149-8

sector economy was expected to continue declining in 2021.[3] This uncertain situation would most likely extend unemployment and limit hiring opportunities, especially for foreign expatriates, in spite of a possible recovery as Gulf industries reopened.

In the Gulf states, the Covid-19 pandemic has therefore taken a particularly heavy toll on low- and semi-skilled migrant labourers, especially coming from South Asia and India.[4] Migrant workers in the GCC economies had already historically subjected to labour rights' violations for a long time. The pandemic has further exposed and exacerbated the exploitation of migrant workers, as evident from the direct layoffs or reductions in working hours owing to lockdowns, as well as the widespread non- or underpayment of wages for work that had been carried out, leading thereby to important earning losses.[5]

The Covid-19 crisis has in many ways also exposed fault lines in the existing Indian migration governance system in dealing with the vulnerabilities experienced by such migrants.[6] These gaps are structural in nature and had been prevailing for a long period, and have remained notwithstanding the improving ties between India and the GCC, especially the UAE and Saudi Arabia.[7] Despite efforts made in recent years at the global level to arrive at a common framework to regulate international labour migration in accordance with international human and labour rights' standards,[8] little progress has been achieved on the issue of wage theft, especially in the context of migrant workers in the Gulf, which are barred from being formally integrated into the socioeconomic structure and legal labour regimes in their countries of destination given both the temporary nature of labour migration and the structural limitations for obtain citizenship or long-term residency in the GCC states. Migrant workers are a special group of employees who are therefore most often not covered by the general protective measures extended by employers and governments in the countries in which they are employed. As a result, a country like India, which has facilitated the movement of migrant workers to the Gulf and has been highly dependent on migrant labour and related remittances, has been struggling to protect these workers during the pandemic.

While there have been some studies about the sanitary, economic and political effects of the coronavirus pandemic in India,[9] and discussion over the internal movement of migrant labourers in India as a consequence of the Covid-19 pandemic,[10] another less discussed issue has been the impact of the health crisis on migrant labourers from India, especially in the GCC. How has the Covid-19 crisis affected the welfare and employment of Indian diaspora communities in the GCC, as well as their ties to their home state? How has the situation impacted India's improving geopolitical ties with some of the GCC states? This chapter intends to examine the effects of the Covid-19 pandemic on foreign expatriate worker communities, especially from South Asia and India, in the Gulf region. This paper aims to look at how the pandemic has exposed the GCC states to structural and new labour governance problems and had a direct spill-over effect on India through remittances, but also owing to the return and reintegration of a significant number of migrant workers. This paper investigates this phenomenon through analysing the complex politics of migration interdependence between India and the GCC that have developed over the last two decades.

In the remainder of this chapter, I first provide a brief historical background of South Asian, and specifically Indian, labour migration to the GCC states. I then discuss how the Covid-19 crisis has impacted South Asian, and specifically Indian, diasporic communities, their employment, their everyday lives in the Gulf, and their ties to their home states. Third, I discuss how the Covid-19 pandemic and the resulting implications for Indian migrant workers have affected India's ties with the GCC states. Finally, I share some concluding thoughts over the future of India's migration governance and foreign policy towards the Gulf region.

Historical Background

The relationship between the GCC and foreign workers, especially from South Asia (India, but also Bangladesh, Nepal, Sri Lanka, and Pakistan) has been one of mutual, if uneven, interdependence. Economic factors have historically been one of the main drivers of migration between South Asia and the Gulf, where millions of migrants emigrate to work. The oil boom in the Gulf countries in the 1970s resulted in a heightened interest for emigration of worker population from South Asia, particularly from India. This development required the service of a large number of foreign workers, as the GCC countries could not provide the indigenous labour supplies. Since the 1970s, the Gulf has therefore positioned itself as a major global destination for migrant workers, following Europe and North America, and 24% of global remittances flow out of the Gulf.[11] In 2019, the Gulf region hosted more than 35 million foreign expatriates employed across various diverse Gulf industries, including construction, hospitality, finance, domestic work, and other service-based sectors.[12] The UAE and Saudi Arabia presently host 70% of the total Gulf foreign expatriate populations, thus acting as vital global labour destination sites for South Asia, with the International Labour Organization (2015) reporting that over 90% of economic migrants from India, Pakistan, and Nepal leave their homes to work in the region. According to the same report, Bangladesh and Nepal send more than 60% of their migrant workers to the GCC region.[13] Although the reliance on foreign labourers is less severe in Saudi Arabia and Oman with under 30% of the foreign labour force, the percentage of expatriates can be ranged from around 90% in Qatar and 70% in the UAE and Kuwait.[14]

Among the South Asian states, India has been the largest supplier of blue-collar and contractual workers in the Gulf region. Indian emigrants in the GCC rose from 1.95 million in 1990 to nearly 9.33 million in 2019 and accounting for 31% of the total migrant population in the region.[15] Tamil Nadu, Andhra Pradesh, Uttar Pradesh, and especially Kerala have been the leading states in India that have met the increasing demand for cheap labour supply to the GCC countries.[16] Indian migrants to the GCC have mainly been low- and semi-skilled workers as they are basically contractual workers in low-paid and inadequately regulated economic sectors, and once their contract expires, migrant workers have to return home.[17] For Indian migrants, the most commonly cited reasons for migration have been wage differences and job opportunities. Most migrants come from the poorer sections of Indian society and their earning potential in Gulf region, even with low education and lack of skills, has been much higher compared to what they get at home and hence perceived as a means for upward economic mobility.[18]

The move of a large number of low-skilled labour migrants has an been implicit (and sometimes explicit) strategy for India to address domestic job creation demand, target poverty levels and stimulate social mobility, offset the cost of social welfare provision, and to generate foreign exchange.[19] The contribution of Indian emigrants in the Gulf to the Indian economy through remittances account for around $35 billion and thereby 1.6 of the national GDP.[20] India has remained the highest remittance receiver in 2018 and attracted about $78.6 billion in remittances, registering a 14% increase over the previous year.[21] Remittances from the Gulf still made up more than half of remittance flows to India.[22] This system has also been beneficial for the migrants who have been able to earn relatively higher incomes and escape the limited socioeconomic opportunities provided by their home states.

However, despite these gains, these migrant workers have often experienced exploitation and violations of their human rights throughout the migration cycle. Labour migrants have had to cope with multiple challenges owing to the vulnerabilities produced by inadequate migration governance in both the sending and receiving states. These challenges and vulnerabilities vary by social class and skill class of labour, by the regularity or irregularity through which the migrant enters the workplace, and by gender, race, and caste. For irregular migrants, work conditions in the GCC states are often precarious and dangerous. Many South Asian migrants operate in gray and unregulated or under-regulated sectors of the labour market. In practice, the temporary sponsorship system allows a precarious type of long-term residence through the regular renewal of contracts and visas. Many expatriates, especially among semi-skilled. and skilled classes of labour, spend their entire working lives in one country and often their children too.[23] In the GCC states, these migrants have had limited access to the appropriate knowledge or networks to support their labour rights. If they are irregular, seeking labour rights support would often result in detention or deportation for violating labour and residency regulations.

The Indian state has been mainly unable to regulate the recruitment industry, which then leave most migrant workers hostage to exploitation by recruitment agencies and employers. For instance, Emigration Clearance Policies (ECR) have been no guarantee of protection for the migrants. The employment visa has remained "a commodity of sale and purchase"[24]; its price level is controlled by recruitment agencies, and this power is exploited and worsened with fraud. The exorbitant recruitment costs endured by low- and semi-skilled migrant workers constitute one of the most challenging problems associated with the India–Gulf migration corridor. Migrants incur costs that are much higher than the legally stipulated limit. Lack of reliable empirical information on recruitment costs has been one of the biggest stumbling blocks in the formulation of effective and sustainable policy responses.

Given the cumbersome regulations in formal recruitment process, many migrants opt for irregular channels to obtain jobs in the Gulf through their own informal (professional, family, local) networks. Many of these migrants have decided to exercise agency by using irregular channels to migrate, thereby opting out of the official governing space and becoming undocumented in India's migration governance systems. Labour migration into GCC countries is also structured by the *kafala* system.[25] Under this system, workers cannot change employment to take up jobs with better working conditions and have to work in those they were originally recruited for. This system also enables employers to confiscate passports of workers and exert significant control over their workers' lives.[26] Consequently, the *kafala* systems creates an excessively unequal power relationship between the employer and the migrant resulting in quite often forced and bonded labour, exploitation and abuse. The system has come under increasing criticism as it has also led to visa trading and promoted irregular migration. *kafala* has been subject to various reforms in Qatar and the UAE in 2020.[27]

As a result, even before the Covid-19 pandemic hit the Gulf economies, the fluctuation of oil prices and changes in Gulf labor policies had led to an increasing scrutiny and condemnation of the treatment of blue-collar and domestic expatriate workers in the GCC, prompting notably a greater attention by the Government of India to diaspora affairs and worker welfare issues. The Indian government has undertaken a wide range of proactive measures to curb exploitation and to ensure the safety and well-being of Indian nationals, notably the setting up of an eMigrate Portal to facilitate the emigration of ECR category of emigrants and to protect them against possible exploitation by unscrupulous recruiters, and to regulate of recruitment industry and agents (MEA Media Center 2017),[28] as well as the setting up of a Minimum Referral Wage to regulate the wages of Indian migrant workers employed in different occupations in ECR countries.[29] Yet, complaints received from and on behalf of migrant workers regarding various forms of abuse, exploitation, and hardship have persisted, notably in light of the unprecedented health and economic challenges posed by the Covid-19 crisis.

In addition, while the role of the Indian state remains of crucial significance, states are not actors operating alone. Rather global governance institutions and governmental actors at the subnational, regional, and international levels all play roles in shaping the governance of migration. Furthermore, non-governmental actors including businesses and activists have also been influential players in the migration governance space.[30] The ways through which sovereignty has been contested and governance is shaped by these various actors and stakeholders is a critical component of how global migration governance occurs in the migration corridor from South Asia to the Gulf. Regulatory choices that occur are not only influenced by the multiplicity of actors operating in this space, but also influence their activities, choices, and advocacy. Recruitment agents, business hiring managers, migrants, and migration advocacy organisations react to regulatory choices by adjusting their activities, lobbying for new regulations, looking for ways of facilitating the continuation of labour migration, and creating new platforms and mechanisms for generating governance change. As a result, the consequences of the Covid-19 crisis, the policy responses and their implications need to be understood through this multi-scalar governance activity in a contested and constantly evolving sovereign space.

Covid-19 and the Indian Diaspora in the Gulf

While the Gulf economies had been facing an economic slowdown caused by the fall in crude oil prices before the spread of Covid-19, the pandemic severely hit the Gulf city economies in 2020 producing a massive pool of unemployed foreign expatriates (including their wives and children) seeking either to return to their home countries or stay in the Gulf region, regardless of their ethnic, gender, and religious backgrounds. The Covid-19 pandemic, and its consequences for migrant workers in terms of wage and income reduction, abrupt loss of employment, and repatriation have further emphasized the vulnerable situation that low- and semi-skilled workers had been experiencing at various phases of the migration cycle.

The Covid-19 crisis affected Indian migrants in two major ways. First, Indian migrants were directly affected by the sanitary crisis as the majority of Covid-19 cases in the Gulf were among foreign migrants. The Covid-19 pandemic significantly impacted not only the Gulf domestic economies, but also the broader state institutions and policies, specifically in the areas of public health, urban policy, employment, and security. Migrants are structurally more vulnerable, owing to inadequate health care, poorer economic conditions, and overcrowded living conditions, which put them at greater risk of infection. Second, as mentioned above, migrant communities were also directly affected by the economic downturn linked to the Covid-19 situation. For 2020, the International Monetary Fund sees economies in the GCC shrinking by 7.6 percent (Barbuscia and Rashad 2020).[31] This has meant massive unemployment, unpaid wages through failing businesses or wage theft, arbitrary detentions or deportations as legal residencies faltered, and a growing need for food handouts. Many Indian migrant workers were initially left stranded, owing to travel bans or unaffordable flight tickets as a result of the lockdowns, travel bans, and limited air traffic options.

In addition, the Covid-19 crisis and the resulting unemployment issues devastated millions deeply dependent on remittances from Gulf migrant workers in India. As indicated above, remittances from the GCC still represented more $35 billion in 2019, of which close to $8 billion was sent to the state of Kerala alone. At least partly as a result of the important remittances and investments made by Kerali immigrants in the Gulf, the state of Kerala is estimated to be about 50% wealthier per head than the national Indian average.[32] Following the economic impact of Covid-19, the World Bank anticipated a 20% fall in remittances to low- and middle-income countries, from 2019's $714 billion (the highest ever) to $572 billion in 2020.[33] This has inevitably affected the traditional and crucial contribution of Indian migrant workers in the Gulf both as a safety valve, to some degree, to address mounting domestic employment problem in India, but also financially to the Indian economy, and especially to the millions of households and Kerala economy which have depended historically on this financial support. Apart from their stabilising effect on India's external reserves, the remittances, particularly from the Gulf region, have had a vital impact in reducing poverty and improving educational and health outcomes of migrant households.

The future for Indian migrant workers in the GCC economies has also been further complicated by the fact some countries like Kuwait have been considering laws limiting foreign workers in the country.[34] If such laws become common across the GCC, they could lead to a situation where many Indian workers could be laid off and sent back home, primarily affecting the sending Indian states of Uttar Pradesh and Bihar, which have been facing high levels of unemployment. Furthermore, taking advantage of these mass repatriation moves have been employers who saw the opportunity to terminate the employment of workers without paying them their legitimate wages, or possible compensation and benefits.[35]

Consequently, since early 2020 many Indian migrant workers and their families have chosen to return to India. Massive repatriation waves are not unprecedented as the welfare of migrants in Gulf labour markets has been affected by a series of Middle Eastern crises in the past decades. During the 1990 Gulf War, nearly 170,000 Indians were evacuated from Kuwait. Similarly, many workers were also left out of a job and returned to India following the 2008–09 global financial crisis.[36] However, the pandemic caused most likely the largest historical return of overseas workers in India. About 300,000 Indians filed for repatriation from the Gulf in May 2020.[37] Of the more than 6 million Indians returned from abroad from all over the world under the Vande Bharata mission, close to 75% migrants were from GCC countries (MEA Media Center 2021).[38]

The challenges for the Indian government has been to first operate the many repatriation flights over a short period and then to assist with the rehabilitation for migrants who return into both the origin society and economy and helping them eventually re-migrate in newly formed migration corridors as the pandemic subsides. While the trend of return migration had

already been growing owing to labour market changes in the Gulf economies, the Covid-19 pandemic has exacerbated the trend. An estimated 20%
of the 9 million Indian population in the Gulf are expected to come back
who are not only migrant workers but also in many cases dependents of
these workers including spouses, children and parents.[39] An additional problem is that many of these Indian migrant workers in the Gulf countries
have also been returning home without months of salary owed to them.

The task of absorbing this sudden return migration has been even more acute
for some Indian states like Kerala.[40] In the case of Kerala, the pandemic exposed
the weakness of a state economy which relied on family members sending
money back home. Of the 307,000 returnees who registered with the state government in August 2020, nearly 55% cited job loss as the reason for their
return.[41] According to some estimates, the aggregate remittance could drop by
$2 billion in 2020.[42] Along with leading to the abrupt return of distressed
migrant workers, the pandemic has also dried up new labour outflows from
India to the GCC states since March 2020. This is the first net decline in the
region since labour migration began to grow considerably in the 1970s. Luckily
for Kerala, there had already been a drop in the number of Keralites moving
from India to the GCC for employment. Consequently, states like Kerala had
begun to prepare for a similar situation (although not this scale) by introducing
training schemes to provide potential emigrant workers with specific skills
(notably training nurses) facilitating migration to Australia and Canada.[43]

In the perspective of mitigating these absorption costs and the impact of
the decrease in remittances, India's External Affairs Minister S. Jaishankar
urged the Gulf countries, in a virtual meeting held with the GCC in
November 2020, to facilitate the return of Indian workers and professionals
who were eager to resume their work following the easing of coronavirus-
related restrictions.[44] In exchange, Jaishankar assured the Gulf nations on
continuing the supply of food, medicines, and of course Covid-19 vaccines
from India (mainly Bahrain and Oman). Indian minister S. Jaishankar further
noted in March 2021 that the "focus of our efforts in the last few months
has now shifted to Indians going back to their usual places of work, study
and domicile," and added that "the largest numbers, not surprisingly, have
gone to the Gulf".[45] Jaishankar also highlighted that the Indian government
had been actively urging Gulf governments "to look sympathetically at the
employment of their citizens as they chart their recovery pathway".[46] Indians
who left the Gulf at the peak of the Covid-19 pandemic have started to
return. Furthermore, despite the economic crisis in the Gulf states, a large
share of Indian migrants expressed their intention to stay, owing partly to
the worsening unemployment problems in India. The structural problems
affecting the low- and semi-skilled labourers who initially moved to the Gulf
economies, such as limited and low-paid opportunities the Indian labour
market, have not have abated and many have still been considering returning to
work in the Gulf economies in spite of the prospects of even more precarious
conditions given the instability in the Gulf economies.

As a result, India faced the twin challenge of absorbing large numbers of its citizens into an already poor domestic job market (and this development disproportionately affected specific states within India), and the potential loss in remittances from the Gulf, which accounts for over half of India's total annual remittances. India seems to have wagered heavily into the possibility for many of these low- and semi-skilled workers to re-migrate from India to the GCC. However, the question is whether the GCC economies will be re-opening to migrant workers over the short term and under similar conditions. Another issue highlighted in the previous section was that... India's existing migration governance framework has been poorly equipped to deal with vulnerabilities encountered by the migrant workers, including the latest Covid-19 crisis-induced insecurities. There are therefore questions over which reforms are required to make India's migration governance structure more cognizant and responsive to the low- and semi-skilled migrant needs and concerns, especially in consideration of anticipated transformations in the post-Covid-19 migration corridor. Any effective Indian response in this space of overlapping sovereignties will also require coordination with the involved GCC states.

Covid-19 and India's Ties with GCC States

Over the last decade, and especially Indian Prime Minister Narendra Modi's tenure, India has pursued a significant policy rapprochement with the GCC states. This rapprochement was driven by structural conditions that justified increased public exchanges with the Gulf States. The GCC have historically a source of more than 60% of India's oil and gas requirements and, therefore, critical to its energy security.[47] The financial value of India's relations with the Gulf countries has also grown over the last decade. While India only represented only 3% of the GCC's total trade in 1992, it represented 11% in 2012. By 2020 Saudi Arabia and the UAE had become India's fourth- and third-largest trade partners.[48] Energy and ties have traditionally dominated India's relations with the Gulf countries but have also been boosted by the existence of a sizeable Indian diaspora. The Gulf states have been home to approximately 8 million Indians who have been contributing about $35 billion in remittances every year and account for close to 1,6% of India's GDP.[49] The strong historical transnational ties between this important diaspora and the populations of specific Indian states (Kerala, Andhra Pradesh, Tamil Nadu) also reinforced the need for Indian leadership to see events and ties with Gulf states as directly affecting the welfare of parts of its society.

The Modi government pushed this burgeoning transactional relationship further and into an economic and political partnership. In an important speech in 2015, India's then Foreign Secretary S. Jaishankar recognised India's "historical presence in the Gulf" but also noted that it had been an "an evolutionary happening that was relatively autonomous of strategic calculations", mostly driven by people and market forces than by "policy".[50]

Jaishankar suggested then that India, rather than being a passive recipient of outcomes build on the "interdependence" and "combination of human and energy connectivity" to further avenues of cooperation and to make India a "credible partner" of actors in the Middle East.[51] As a result, Modi's multiple and repeated visits to the Gulf countries have been an effort to build on and consolidate existing economic ties. Modi focused his attention on the Gulf with the clear goal of strengthening government-to-government ties by building on existing business-to-business contacts at the highest levels. One specific objective was also to encourage Gulf sovereign wealth funds to invest in Modi's ambitious infrastructure and manufacturing plans at home. From 2015 to 2019 the UAE and Saudi Arabia pledged a combined total of $170 billion to help India develop its infrastructure in the energy and industrial sectors.[52] Modi even chose the UAE as his first Middle East visit in August 2015, but he also visited Saudi Arabia, Iran and Qatar in 2016, as well as the UAE again in 2018 and 2019. During his second visit to the UAE, Modi was rewarded the Order of Zayed, the UAE's highest civil decoration, in recognition of his role in improving ties between the two countries. Modi not only travelled again to Saudi Arabia, but also to Oman, and Bahrain in a wide outreach to the Gulf states. All these trips were reciprocated by visits of Gulf dignitaries to New Delhi during the same time period.

The diplomatic efforts of the last few years have also had geopolitical gains, notably by serving to dilute Pakistan's traditionally strong influence among the Gulf states. Saudi Arabia and the UAE no longer view ties with India and Pakistan as a zero-sum game. While both of these Gulf states maintain their political ties with Pakistan, they prioritize investments in India. This subtle shift has had a geopolitical effect, as both Gulf states have toned down their rhetoric condemning India on its policy toward Kashmir, a region disputed between India and Pakistan. For example, the timing of the announcement of Saudi Aramco's $15 billion investment in India in August 2019, one week after New Delhi's controversial move to revoke Kashmir's special status, seemed like a gesture indicating that Saudi Arabia was no longer willing to let the Kashmir issue be an obstacle to better ties with India.[53] Similarly, the UAE also announced that it viewed India's Kashmir decision as "an internal matter".[54]

The Modi government's active diplomatic outreach to the Gulf states had until recently shied away from commenting on the situation of its low- and semi-skilled labourers based in the GCC states. Whereas discussions over the labour and human rights of Indian expatriate workers had traditionally hounded India's ties with some Gulf states, the Indian diaspora in the Middle East was framed in a new light by both Jaishankar and Modi in a series of statements between 2015 and 2020. In this new rhetoric, the diaspora was presented as an important actor and factor in facilitating better understanding and ties between India and the Gulf. A series of policy initiatives mentioned above like the eMigrate system in 2015 were also launched by the Indian government to ensure safe migration to the Gulf, to strengthen the outreach initiatives of Indian Gulf embassies, and to opening new grievance redressal windows for expatriate workers.[55] In addition, India and the UAE had also negotiated easing of travel and work-related migration formalities. These related to e-visa arrangements for migrant workers from India and multiple entry visas for visitors from the UAE.[56]

However, the early phase of the Covid-19 pandemic has led to India's Muslim community facing online and physical assaults—incidents in which members of the ruling Bharatiya Janata Party (BJP) were also implicated.[57] These attacks came in the wake of news that an Islamic sect, the Tablighi Jamaat, held a large annual meeting in New Delhi's Nizamuddin district in early March, right as countries were beginning to restrict public gatherings to prevent the virus's spread. With nearly 3,000 pilgrims from over a dozen countries packed in cramped quarters, the coronavirus spread rapidly; the assembly was identified as a major source of infections in India.[58] The following statements expressing concerns over the BJP's treatment of Indian Muslims, notably from the OIC led India's minister for external affairs, Jaishankar, to promptly placate concerns of his counterparts in the UAE, Qatar, Oman and Saudi Arabia by reaffirming that the government would continue to provide food suppliers to Indian Muslims during the holy month of Ramadan and would make any medical treatment available to fight the pandemic.[59]

Hence, the Covid-19 crisis and its consequences on domestic communal relations in India threatened to disrupt India's ties with the Gulf states, at a time when India also had to negotiate repatriation efforts of migrant workers in the Gulf, the issue of unpaid wages from Gulf employers, and the possibility of re-migration in a post-Covid-19 situation. Given the increasing *migration interdependence* between India and some GCC states like the UAE and Qatar, India has been increasingly conscious of both the opportunities and constraints the presence of migrants can create to further diplomatic and economic ties.[60] While India is strongly dependent on remittances and other economic benefits coming from its diaspora in the Gulf, the GCC states have also been pushing for increased non-oil trade with an emerging market like India,[61] as well as the labour supply despite the efforts of GCC states to restrict and reduce the share of migrants in their total populations. As a result, the issue of allowing of Indian workers to return to their destination countries is most likely to be taken up in the context of these high-level trade negotiations.

Conclusion

The Covid-19 pandemic has accelerated many inherent problems linked to the labour-intensive character of the GCC economies that have had a direct spillover effect on India. While some actors in India, like the state of Kerala, had begun to gradually adapt to reverse migration from labourers in the Gulf, the acceleration of this trend, along with the falling GDP growth in

India that had preceded the Covid-19 pandemic, further highlighted the vulnerability of Indian migrant workers and the gaps in migration governance structure.

While the slow economic reopening has helped some Gulf-based companies to recover slightly, the vast majority have still been struggling. This lagged and uneven recovery has had severe adverse effects on the quantity and quality of employment opportunities in the Gulf private sector. In particular, Gulf government's limited fiscal budget could also impact their existing infrastructure projects, which significantly recruited foreign expatriates. For example, Saudi Arabia has already cut $8 billion from its Vision 2030 to cope with its fiscal budget constraints.[62] Other Gulf countries like Kuwait, Bahrain, and Oman also restructured their national fiscal budgets to maintain financial liquidity in 2021.[63]

In addition, Gulf employment is likely to remain limited in the long run, except in specific critical sectors like health, food, and logistics. To a large extent, the labour dependence for various vital industries (i.e. hospitality, aviation, construction) will likely generate unemployment as Gulf-companies have begun to cut operational costs and maintain liquidity as Gulf economy and businesses try to recover in the short run. Localization policies have also intensified, specifically in Oman's and Kuwait's private sectors. The UAE and Saudi Arabian governments, however, have not strongly promulgated localization policies but their socioeconomic policies (UAE's increase of government fees related to work permits for instance) could indirectly trigger the outflow of foreign expatriates living and working in the Gulf.[64] As a result, Gulf states will also continue to impose restrictive and authoritative labour market protectionism and policing to control the spread of Covid-19, and its impact on their economies.

These restrictive employment policies in the Gulf will likely lead to more illegal migration. With limited employment and economic prospects in India, and perceived weak governance responses to the Covid-19-induced crisis, combined with large financial responsibilities to support their families, foreign expatriates will be encouraged to try to move back or to stay in the Gulf countries irrespective of their immigration status, owing to potential opportunities to earn income in the Gulf formal or informal markets. The wage differential dimension of the Gulf-sending country destinations is likely to continuing playing a critical role on foreign expatriates' micro-decisions to stay in the Gulf, while simultaneously hoping for the future economic recovery of the Gulf economy.

Finally, the recent migration trends and the consequences of the economic crisis wrought by the Covid-19 pandemic will most likely have a lasting impact on India's policies towards the Gulf. The imperative for Indian policymakers to address will be to facilitate re-migration of low- and semi-skilled migration to the GCC states but also to ensure that this does not happen via illegal means or through high recruitment costs borne by the individual migrants. The existing air travel bubble arrangements between India and GCC countries based on prescribed travel and health protocols must be used effectively to enable the journeys of those willing to go back. There is also a strong need to restructure the Emigration Act of 1983 to adjust it to the changing migration landscape and to ensure it responds effectively to migrant's needs. The vulnerabilities that migrant workers often encounter in destination countries, such as violation of the provisions of the agreed employment contracts, arise because of the asymmetry in information between the employer and the intending emigrant. The law must have clear provisions to ensure that the migrant workers obtain all relevant information about the terms of employment from the employer or recruiting agencies. In this regard, the Emigration Bill 2021, which is currently at the consultation stage with all stakeholders, could help establish a comprehensive emigration framework with adequate opportunities for migration and mobility and safeguards against exploitation of Indian workers abroad.

Studies of India's migration towards the GCC have demonstrated that the bulk of initiative is still individual-driven rather than the outcome of an institutionalised migration governance system.[65] There is therefore an urgent need for states like India, with a long history of migration links with the Gulf, but also improving political and economic ties with the GCC states, to promote and institutionalise labour migration in its bilateral ties with the relevant regional actors, notably to ensure skill certification and accreditation systems in the destination countries, as well as discussions over minimum wages and legal and social coverage. Furthermore, as return migration is an inherent aspect of the India-Gulf migration flows, given the temporary nature of labour migrant employment, this question needs to be given further attention in bilateral negotiations over Labour Employment and Cooperation Agreements, especially in light of the distressed situations of retuning migrants during the ongoing pandemic. Such consultations can ensure the sustainability of this migration corridor for all stakeholders.

Notes

1 Neha Bhatia, 'IMF forecasts a 7.1 per cent drop in GCC's GDP', *Middle East Business Intelligence*, July 14, 2020. Available at: www.meed.com/imf-projects-71-p er-cent-drop-in-gccs-gdp [Last accessed September 30, 2021].

2 Gulf Health Council, 'The GCC Countries Face COVID19: A Report which Clarifies the Efforts of the Gulf Cooperation Council Countries to Stop the Spread of COVID19 and Limit the Expected Negative Economic Effects on the Countries of the Gulf Region', August 10, 2020. Available at http://ghc.sa/ar- sa/ Documents/The%20GCC%20Countries%20Face%20COVID-19.pdf [Last accessed September 30, 2021].

3 Bhatia, 'IMF forecasts a 7.1 per cent drop in GCC's GDP'.

4 Joanna Slater, Kareem Fahim and Katie McQue, 'Migration, in Reverse,' *Washington Post*, October 1, 2020. Available at: www.washingtonpost.com/graphics/2020/ world/coronavirus-migration-trends-gulf-states-india/?itid=sf_world [Last accessed September 30, 2021].

5 Manolo I. Abella, 'Labour Migration Policy Dilemmas in the Wake of COVID-19', *International Migration*, 58, no. 4 (2020). Available at: https://doi.org/10.1111/imig.

12746 [Last accessed September 30, 2021]; International Labour Office, 'Labour Migration' (2020). Available at: www.ilo.org/beirut/areasofwork/labour-migration/lang–en/index.htm [Last accessed September 30, 2021]; World Bank, 'Potential Responses to the COVID-19 Outbreak in Support of Migrant Workers', June 19, 2020. World Bank Group. Available at: https://openknowledge.worldbank.org/handle/10986/33625 [Last accessed September 30, 2021],

6   Crystal Ennis and Nicolas Blarel, eds, *The South Asia to Gulf Migration Governance Complex* (Bristol: Bristol University Press, 2022).

7   Nicolas Blarel, 'Modi looks West? Assessing change and continuity in India's Middle East policy since 2014', *International Politics* (2021). Available at: https://doi.org/10.1057/s41311-021-00314-3 [Last accessed September 30, 2021].

8   Laura Foley and Nicola Piper, 'Returning home empty handed: Examining how COVID-19 exacerbates the non-payment of temporary migrant workers' wages', *Global Social Policy* (2021). Available at: https://doi.org/10.1177/14680181211012958 [Last accessed September 30, 2021].

9   Adam M. Auerbach and Tariq Thachil, 'How does COVID-19 affect urban slums? Evidence from settlement leaders in India', *World Development*, 140 (2021). Available at: https://doi.org/10.1016/j.worlddev.2020.105304 [Last accessed September 30, 2021]; Niladri Chatterjee, Zaad Mahmood, and Eleonor Marcussen, 'Politics of Vaccine Nationalism in India: Global and Domestic Implications', Forum for Development Studies 48, no. 2 (2021): 357–369; Anwesha Dutta and Harry W. Fischer, 'The local governance of COVID-19: Disease prevention and social security in rural India', *World Development*, 138 (2021). Available at: https://doi.org/10.1016/j.worlddev.2020.105234 [Last accessed September 30, 2021]; Alf Gunvald Nilsen, 'India's pandemic: spectacle, social murder and authoritarian politics in a lockdown nation', *Globalizations* (2021). Available at: https://doi.org/10.1080/14747731.2021.1935019 [Last accessed September 30, 2021]; Amit Prakash, 'Introduction to a special issue of India Review: Reflections on Politics and Policy for a post-COVID-19 Era: Analysing Continuities and Fractures through the First Wave of 2020', *India Review*, 20, no. 2 (2021): 97–103; Pradeep Taneja and Azad Singh Bali, 'India's domestic and foreign policy responses to COVID-19', *The Round Table*, 110, no. 1 (2021): 46–61.

10   Rajiv Ranjan, 'Impact of COVID-19 on Migrant Labourers of India and China', *Critical Sociology*, 47, no. 4–5 (2021): 721–726; Aayesha Saxena, '(Re)visiting the legitimacy of the state: COVID-19 and the migrant labor in India', *India Review*, 20, no. 2 (2021): 194–212.

11   World Bank, 'Potential Responses to the COVID-19 Outbreak'.

12   International Labour Office (ILO), *ILO Global Estimates on International Migrant Workers – Results and Methodology*, 2nd ed. (Geneva: ILO, n.d.). Available at: www.ilo.org/wcmsp5/groups/public/—dgreports/—dcomm/—publ/documents/publication/wcms_652001.pdf [Last accessed September 30, 2021].

13   International Labour Organization (ILO), *Labour Market Trends Analysis and Labour Migration from South Asia to Gulf Cooperation Council Countries, India and Malaysia* (Eschborn and Geneva: Deutsche Gesellschaft für Internationale Zusammenarbeit GmbH and International Labour Organization, 2015), 6. Available online: www.ilo.org/wcmsp5/groups/public/—ed_protect/—protrav/—migrant/documents/publication/wcms_378239.pdf [Last accessed September 30, 2021].

14   S. Irudaya Rajan and Prem Saxena, eds, *India's Low-Skilled Migration to the Middle East: Policies, Politics and Challenges* (Singapore: Palgrave Macmillan, 2019).

15   UNDESA, *International Migrant Stock 2019* (New York: United Nations Department of Economic and Social Affairs, 2019).

16   S. Irudaya Rajan, 'Demography of Gulf Region' in Mehdi Chowdhury and S. Iduraya. Rajan, eds, *South Asian Migration in the Gulf* (Basingstoke: Palgrave Macmillan, 2018), 35–59.

17 K. C. Zachariah and S. Idurayan Rajan. *Emigration in Kerala: End of an Era* (Cochin: Nalanda Books, 2018).

18 The data relating to low- and semi-skilled labour migration to the GCC has been captured by emigration clearances, a statutory requirement for those with emigration check required (ECR) passports, generally issued to Indian citizens with an educational attainment below 10th standard migrating to 18 labelled ECR countries, which includes all the GCC countries. See Ministry of External Affairs (MEA), 'Transcript of Media Briefing on E-Migrate', MEA Media Center, January 19, 2017. Available at: https://mea.gov.in/media-briefings.htm?dtl/27958 [Last accessed September 30, 2021]. In fact, more than 95% of these clearances obtained during 2010–19 were for migrants to the GCC countries. See S.K. Sasikumar, 'India–Gulf Labour Migration in the Aftermath of the COVID-19 Pandemic', *Economic and Political Weekly*, 56, no. 34 (2021): 22–26.

19 S. Krishna Kumar and S. Irudaya Rajan, *Emigration in 21st-Century India: Governance, Legislation, Institutions* (New Delhi: Routledge, 2014).

20 World Bank-KNOMAD, 'Migration and Remittances: Recent Developments and Outlook- Special Topic: Financing for Development', *Migration and Development Brief*, 24, April 2015. Available online: www.knomad.org/publication/migration-and-development-brief-24 [Last accessed September 30, 2021].

21 World Bank-KNOMAD, 'Migration and Remittances: Recent Developments and Outlook- Special Topic: Financing for Development', *Migration and Development Brief*, 31, April 2019. Available online: www.knomad.org/publication/migration-and-development-brief-31 [Last accessed September 30, 2021].

22 Reserve Bank of India, 'Globalising People: India's Inward Remittances', *RBI Bulletin*, 72, no.11 (2018): 45–56; World Bank-KNOMAD, 'COVID-19 Crisis through a Migration Lens', *Migration and Development Brief*, 32, April 2020. Available at: www.worldbank.org/en/topic/socialprotection/publication/COVID-19-crisis-through-a-migration-lens [Last accessed September 30, 2021].

23 Michael C. Ewers and Ryan Dicce, 'Expatriate Labour Markets in Rapidly Globalising Cities: Reproducing the Migrant Division of Labour in Abu Dhabi and Dubai', *Journal of Ethnic and Migration Studies*, 42, no. 15 (2016): 2439–58; Neha Vora, *Impossible Citizens: Dubai's Indian Diaspora* (Durham: Duke University Press, 2013).

24 Irudaya S. Rajan, V.J. Varghese and M.S. Jayakumar, *Dreaming Mobility and Buying Vulnerability* (New Delhi: Routledge, 2011), 58.

25 *Kafala* comes from the Arabic root k-f-l – to sponsor. The *kafeel* is the individual sponsor. *Kafala* is a sponsorship system, akin to guest worker programmes. Migrants' work and residency are tied to their sponsor, an individual or company. For more, see James Sater, 'Citizenship and migration in Arab Gulf Monarchies', *Citizenship Studies*, 18, no. 3–4 (2014): 292–302.

26 The use of the term *"kafala* system" in English give the impression that it is a uniform system that is applied across the Gulf. However, the regulations which shape immigration into each GCC countries differs and is subject to independent regulatory amendments.

27 Noha Aboueldahab, 'Social protection, not just legal protection: Migrant laborers in the Gulf', *Brookings Doha Center Report*, August 23, 2021. Available at: www.brookings.edu/research/social-protection-not-just-legal-protection-migrant-laborers-in-the-gulf [Last accessed September 30, 2021].

28 MEA, 'Transcript of Media Briefing on E-Migrate'.

29 Nidhi Menon and Rohini Mitra, 'How India's move to reduce minimum referral wages could hurt its workers in the Gulf', Scroll.in, June 23, 2021. Available at: https://scroll.in/article/997850/how-indias-move-to-reduce-minimum-referral-wages-could-hurt-its-workers-in-the-gulf [Last accessed September 30, 2021].

30 Ennis and Blarel, *The South Asia to Gulf Migration Governance Complex*.

31 Davide Barbuscia and Marwa Rashad, 'Gulf economies to shrink by 7.6% this year, IMF says', Reuters June 30, 2020. Available at: www.reuters.com/article/us-gulf-economy-imf-idUSKBN2411RS [Last accessed September 30, 2021].

32 *The Economist*, 'Like Manna from Heaven: How a Torrent of Money from Workers Abroad Reshapes an Economy', September 5, 2015. Available at: www.economist.com/finance-and-economics/2015/09/03/like-manna-from-heaven [Last accessed September 30, 2021].

33 World Bank-KNOMAD, 'COVID-19 Crisis through a Migration Lens'.

34 Kapil Kajal, 'Kuwaiti Dream of Cutting Foreign Workers Threatens Indians Most', Nikkei Asia. August 13, 2020. Available at: https://asia.nikkei.com/Politics/International-relations/Kuwaiti-dream-of-cutting-foreign-workers-threatens-Indians-most [Last accessed September 30, 2021].

35 S.R. Praveen, ''Wage Theft,' a Bane of Gulf Returnees.' *The Hindu*, July 30, 2021. Available at: www.thehindu.com/news/national/kerala/wage-theft-a-bane-of-gulf-returnees/article35623859.ece [Last accessed September 30, 2021].

36 S. Irudaya Rajan, 'The Crisis of Gulf Migration' in Cecilia Menjivar, Marie Ruiz, and Immanuel Ness, eds, *The Oxford Handbook of Migration Crises* (New York: Oxford University Press, 2019), 849–868.

37 Rezaul H. Laskar, 'Over 300,000 Indians register to return from Gulf region, only those with 'compelling reasons' to be brought back in first phase', *Hindustan Times*, May 5, 2020. Available at: www.hindustantimes.com/india-news/over-300-000-indians-register-to-return-from-gulf-region-only-those-with-compelling-reasons-to-be-brought-back-in-first-phase/story-A4qNuaOzlJVQnIclILXxgO.html [Last accessed September 30, 2021].

38 Ministry of External Affairs, 'Rajya Sabha Question NO.188 Indian Workers Returning from Gulf Countries', MEA Media Center, August 5, 2021. Available at: www.mea.gov.in/rajya-sabha.htm?dtl/34119/QUESTION+NO188+INDIAN+WORKERS+RETURNING+FROM+GULF+COUNTRIES [Last accessed September 30, 2021].

39 S. Irudaya Rajan and Ginu Zacharia Oommen, 'The Future of Asian Migration to the Gulf' in S. Irudaya Rajan and Ginu Zacharia Oommen, eds, Asianization of Migrant Workers in the Gulf Countries (Singapore: Springer, 2020), 281–286.

40 but also others as in recent years, the northern states of Uttar Pradesh and Bihar (among the poorest states in India) accounted for nearly half of the emigration clearances issued, see MEA, 'Transcript of Media Briefing on E-Migrate'.

41 Sasikumar, 'India–Gulf Labour Migration'.

42 Manolo I. Abella and S. K. Sasikumar, 'Estimating Earnings Losses of Migrant Workers Due to COVID-19', *Indian Journal of Labour Economics*, 63 (2020): 921–39.

43 Margaret Walton-Roberts, 'International Migration of Health Professionals and the Marketization and Privatization of Health Education in India: From Push-Pull to Global Political Economy', *Social Science and Medicine*, 124 (2015): 374–382.

44 Rezaul H. Laskar, ''Facilitate return of Indian workers, professionals': Jaishankar tells Gulf states', *Hindustan Times*, November 3, 2020. Available at: www.hindustantimes.com/india-news/facilitate-return-of-indian-workers-professionals-jaishankar-tells-gulf-states/story-LV5NnNOZgTWOnfFZnaqvYK.html [Last accessed September 30, 2021].

45 The Hindu, 'Parliament Proceedings | Government to expand air bubble option with more countries: Jaishankar', *The Hindu*, March 15, 2021. Available at: www.thehindu.com/news/national/parliament-proceedings-45-million-indians-brought-back-home-during-pandemic-jaishankar/article34074940.ece [Last accessed September 30, 2021].

46 Ibid.

47 Press Trust of India, 'India's oil import from Middle East rises to 59%', Livemint, April 25, 2016. Available at: www.livemint.com/Industry/9n0jzqdP24Pm

BB13sjRYQJ/Indias-oil-import-from-Middle-East-rises-to-59.html [Last accessed September 30, 2021].

48 Sanjay Pulipaka and Mohit Musaddi, 'Power shifts and re-calibrations: India and the Gulf', *The Economic Times*, February 14, 2020. Available at: https://econom ictimes.indiatimes.com/blogs/et-commentary/power-shifts-and-re-calibrations-india -and-the-gulf/ [Last accessed September 30, 2021].

49 Rukmini Shrinivasan, 'India was the top recipient of remittances worldwide in 2018', *The Economic Times*, July 20, 2019. Available at: https://economictimes.india times.com/nri/forex-and-remittance/india-was-the-top-recipient-of-remittances-world wide-in-2018/articleshow/70310386.cms?from=mdr [Last accessed September 30, 2021].

50 S. Jaishankar. 'Speech by Foreign Secretary at Raisina Dialogue in New Delhi', Minis-try of External Affairs, Government of India, March 2, 2015. Available at: https://mea. gov.in/Speeches-Statements.htm?dtl/26433/Speech_by_Foreign_Secretary_at_Raisina_ Dialogue_in_New_Delhi_March_2_2015 [Last accessed September 30, 2021].

51 Ibid.

52 Jennifer Gnana, 'Planned Aramco-Adnoc refinery in India to cost $70bn', *The National*, November 28, 2019. Available at: www.thenationalnews.com/business/ energy/planned-aramco-adnoc-refinery-in-india-to-cost-70bn-1.943759 [Last acces-sed September 30, 2021].

53 Vindu Goel, 'As Saudis and Indians Grow Closer, a $15 Billion Deal Blooms', *The New York Times*, August 12, 2019. Available at: www.nytimes.com/2019/08/12/busi ness/reliance-india-saudi-aramco-oil.html [Last accessed September 30, 2021].

54 Geeta Mohan, 'UAE backs India on Article 370, says Kashmir its internal matter', *India Today*, August 6, 2019. Available at: www.indiatoday.in/india/ story/article-370-jammu-kashmir-uae-ambassador-dr-al-banna-1577918-2019-08-06 [Last accessed September 30, 2021].

55 Seema Gaur, 'Policies for Protection of Indian Migrant Workers in Middle East' in S. Irudaya Rajan, and Prem Saxena, eds, *India's Low-Skilled Migration to the Middle East: Policies, Politics and Challenges* (Singapore: Palgrave Macmillan, 2019), 138–143.

56 Arabinda Acharya, 'COVID-19: A Testing Time for UAE–India Relations? A Perspective from Abu Dhabi', *Strategic Analysis*, 44, no. 3 (2020): 259–268.

57 Sumit Ganguly and Nicolas Blarel, 'Why Gulf States Are Backtracking on India. Foreign Policy', *Foreign Policy*, May 5, 2020. Available at: https://foreignpolicy. com/2020/05/05/gulf-states-backtracking-india [Last accessed September 30, 2021].

58 Akash Bisht and Sadiq Naqvi, 'How Tablighi Jamaat Event Became India's Worst Coronavirus Vector', Al Jazeera. April 7. Available at: www.aljazeera.com/news/ 2020/4/7/how-tablighi-jamaat-event-became-indias-worst-coronavirus-vector [Last accessed September 30, 2021].

59 Jyoti Malhotra, 'As Gulf calls for an 'India without Islamophobia,' Jaishankar works the phones.' *The Print*, April 28, 2020. Available at: https://theprint.in/op inion/global-print/gulf-calls-india-without-islamophobia-jaishankar-works-phones/ 410159/ [Last accessed September 30, 2021].

60 Gerasimos Tsourapas, 'Labor Migrants as Political Leverage: Migration Inter-dependence and Coercion in the Mediterranean', *International Studies Quarterly*, 62, no. 2 (2018): 383–395.

61 Sylvia Westall and Shruti Srivastava, 'UAE, India Aim to Double Trade to $100 Billion in Five Years', Bloomberg, September 21, 2021. Available at: www.bloomberg.com/news/articles/2021-09-22/uae-seeks-100-billion-india-trade-a s-it-deepens-ties?utm_campaign=socialflow-organic&utm_source=twitter&utm_ content=middleeast&utm_medium=social [Last accessed September 30, 2021].

62 Vivan Nereim, 'Saudi Arabia 'Vision 2030' Plan Cut by $8 Billion, Okaz Reports', Bloomberg, May 12, 2020. Available at: www.bloomberg.com/news/a

rticles/2020-05-12/saudi-arabia-vision-2030-plan-cut-by-8-billion-okaz-reports [Last accessed February 3, 2022].

63 World Bank, 'COVID-19 Pandemic and the Road to Diversification', *Gulf Economic Update*, 6, August 2021. Available at: https://documents1.worldbank.org/curated/en/748461627924058675/pdf/Gulf-Economic-Update-COVID-19-Pandemic-and-the-Road-to-Diversification.pdf [Last accessed September 30, 2021].

64 Raajeshwari Ashok, Ramadan Al Sherbini, and Yasmena Al Mulla, 'Jobs in the Gulf: Saudi Arabia, Kuwait, Oman seek workforce of nationals', *Gulf News*, February 3, 2021. Available at: https://gulfnews.com/special-reports/jobs-in-the-gulf-saudi-arabia-kuwait-oman-seek-workforce-of-nationals-1.76925766 [Last accessed September 30, 2021].

65 Ennis and Blarel, *The South Asia to Gulf Migration Governance Complex*.

9 India and the Institutional Politics of Global Governance Post-Covid-19

Karthik Nachiappan

Introduction

There is broad consensus that global governance is under stress. Debates about whether the current international order is fit for purpose given the pressures and constraints imposed by shifts in the balance of power have become common. The purported weakening of US hegemony and the ascent of rising powers like China and India have ostensibly weakened an already enfeebled system. Covid-19 arrived at this juncture. This chapter covers India's response and attitudes toward two institutional shifts in global governance that were present before and have only hastened after Covid-19. This chapter argues that the rise of minilateral initiatives and emergence and clout of non-state actors like the Gates Foundation within international rule-making has left India flatfooted and unsettled given its cross-cutting economic interests that compel it to support causes that advance interests, engage cautiously or disengage when interests are undermined. Simply put, India's economic interests are inflecting how and where India chooses to multilaterally engage and how.

Fundamentally, India has adjusted to these structural and institutional shifts in global governance that have accelerated, owing to Covid-19, relative to where its security and economic interests and priorities lie. US-Chinese tensions before and since Covid-19 has precipitated a range of security minilaterals including the Quadrilateral Security Dialogue (Quad) that India has openly endorsed and participated in. These initiatives allow India to pool their resources and capabilities with like-minded partners to enhance their collective security in an increasingly fractious regional landscape. But India has, thus far, remained cautious and non-committal when negotiating issues like digital trade, data, 5G and artificial intelligence at various minilateral frameworks given concerns around how engagement will affect India's domestic economic transition that is rapidly digitizing. At these frameworks, Indian officials cannot project their development priorities nor can they bandwagon with other developing countries to advance and protect their interests. The narrow, purposeful and action-oriented nature of such minilateral frameworks makes it harder for countries like India with specific

DOI: 10.4324/9781003248149-9

economic trajectories and interests to shape and exploit their agenda. India, as a result, has appeared reluctant to join and work with economic minilateral frameworks. On global health cooperation, India's focus and agenda vis-a-vis vaccines, particularly vaccine equity, has been constrained by the interests of domestic pharma manufacturers like the Serum Institute who prefer to enter commercial agreements with the Indian government, bilaterally with other countries and multilateral partners like COVAX.

The chapter proceeds as follows. The first section covers the first shift within global governance - the rise of minilateralism, how Covid-19 has hastened this form of international rule-making and India's behaviour vis-a-vis security and economic minilateral initiatives, particularly frameworks focusing on maritime security, trade, technology and digital issues. The second section focuses on the rise and growing clout of non-state actors, specifically the Bill and Melinda Gates Foundation, over global health organizations and policy making. Covid-19 has made the Gates Foundation indispensable through its efforts to cobble together a multilateral response to Covid-19 through vaccine development and its ongoing support to Indian pharma companies like the Serum Institute and Bharat Biotech. The Gates Foundation's neoliberal approach to global health and vaccine development has constrained India, which has appeared timid in raising concerns of vaccine equity at the World Health Organization (WHO), given the interests of its domestic vaccine manufacturers. The conclusion looks ahead to what India could do in the future to better manage these institutional shifts in global governance as its own economic interests evolve.

Security Minilateralism

Covid-19 has hastened the development and use of minilateral and plurilateral frameworks to address policy challenges in the international order. Minilaterals are informal initiatives designed to tackle and address a 'specific threat, contingency or security issue' among three or more countries whose interests converge when it comes to managing and addressing that issue (Tirkey, 2021). Such initiatives are differentiated by their small size, disaggregated scope, bottom-up focus, voluntary participation, non-binding commitments and ad hoc nature. Minilaterals are coalitions driven by interests, willingness and purpose. Countries like India are now increasingly having collective discussions on salient economic and security issues at such informal venues. Such initiatives are fundamentally exclusive, driven by a need to include and convene countries, likely in the same region, that have a motivation to address a specific policy problem like climate change, maritime security or digital protectionism; in other words, purpose and action are critical for minilateral meetings unlike multilateral discussions, which often prioritize process, deliberation and inclusion (Patrick, 2015).

There are two reasons for this trend. First, the Covid-19 pandemic has sensitized countries to the importance of protecting domestic economic trajectories and interests, especially from rivals and competitors that appear as threats. Specifically, Covid-19 has accelerated pre-existing geopolitical trends— the marked decline in American interest toward multilateralism and international organizations and the US-Chinese rivalry that now has a perceptible multilateral manifestation. Sino-US tensions are threatening existing global institutions and rules through 'the exercise of raw power' with each side jostling for control of global markets and resources (Woods, 2021). Since the Obama administration, Washington has eschewed signing multilateral trade and security agreements and largely preferred unilateralism or minilateralism as witnessed through the initial interest toward the Trans-Pacific Partnership (TPP). Beijing has assiduously attempted to establish its own geopolitical sphere through bilateral trade, investment and infrastructure packages under its Belt and Road Initiative (Johnston, 2019). Within the UN, China has countered America's multilateral disdain with a concerted effort to deepen its footprint at multilateral discussions, demonstrated by its activities at the UN Human Rights Council where countries across the developing world supported Beijing on human rights issues in Hong Kong, Xinjiang and Tibet (Piccone, 2021). Rising US-Chinese tensions risks rendering UN agencies, including WHO and COP-26 as mere pawns whose purpose and focus could be sacrificed at the altar of great power competition.

The spread of the coronavirus has intensified and exacerbated existing multilateral tensions. Recently, the WHO was pilloried over its relationship with China that purportedly dented its response to Covid-19 after the initial outbreak (World Health Organization, 2020). Critics contend that Beijing hoodwinked the WHO, particularly with respect to getting and sharing information that could help resolve questions behind the origins of the coronavirus (Mitchell, 2020). The pandemic has raised fundamental doubts over whether China can be a trusted multilateral stakeholder which has galvanized some countries to look for other alternatives to address transboundary problems. Indeed, capacity constraints, specifically defense and surveillance, in South and Southeast Asian countries to monitor and manage a restive maritime space has precipitated minilateral security partnerships (Haruko, 2020). China also continues to have territorial disputes with several Indo-Pacific countries; and despite the crises wrought by the Covid-19 pandemic, Beijing has attempted to resolve these quarrels unilaterally through the establishment of an air-defense identification zone and related measures that constrain navigation across the South China Sea (Singh, 2020). The inability to restrain China's behaviour has compelled countries to pool their capabilities and withstand Chinese power. Covid-19 has sharpened and extended US-Chinese rivalry particularly over control over legitimacy in the Indo-Pacific and across other international organizations that decide the rules of the international order.

India has not adapted nimbly enough to this emergent minilateral reality and landscape, particularly vis-à-vis minilateral economic initiatives, as its economic interests appear divided between that of developing and developed countries. To be sure, India appears more comfortable to engage in various security minilaterals, like the Quad and other trilaterals, albeit cautiously. Initially, India had inhibitions over minilateral frameworks given bilateral security concerns with China, especially across the northern border. It appears China's aggressive behaviour before and especially since June 2020 has nudged India forward on the minilateral path. Beijing's recent assertiveness has allowed India and regional partners like Australia and Japan to work through mechanisms like the Quad to solidify deterrence and signal their collective resolve against Beijing.

Quad aside, India is also connected through a litany of trilateral initiatives like India-France-Australia, Australia-Japan-India, Japan-US-India, Australia-India-Indonesia, and India-Italy-Japan to foster regional security (Singh and Teo, 2020). Two specific trilaterals appear salient post Covid-19 outbreak given the need to strengthen maritime security: India-France-Australia and India-Australia-Indonesia (Rajagopalan, 2021). In September 2020 the India-France-Australia trilateral convened virtually to take stock on rising threats across the 'maritime global commons' and how these can be addressed by partnering with existing partners like ASEAN, IORA, and Indian Ocean Commission. After initial meetings in 2018 and 2019, the India-Australia-Indonesia trilateral convened virtually in September 2020 to discuss maritime matters, specifically 'development assistance programs and HADR efforts' (Tillett and Connors, 2020).

Such minilaterals allow middle powers like India, Australia, Indonesia, Japan, and France to use convergences to deepen the institutional landscape governing regional security and growth as questions around the credibility and longevity of the US alliance system linger (Tow, 2020). Capacity constraints also matter with Covid-19 battering economic growth potentials across the region, especially India that is yet to fully revive its economy. Uncertainty around Washington's security role and presence has compelled middle powers to forge closer ties to manage and neutralize extant security and economic concerns efficiently. As Aarshi Tirkey points out, the dramatic improvement of communications technologies including through the internet, independent of Covid-19, which precipitated virtual summits and discussions, could have increased the use and utility of minilaterals that require little institutional support to function (Tirkey, 2021). Although the advent of technologies has facilitated such meetings, their effects on the scope of international cooperation remain questionable even as they appear to be altering the nature and frequency of multilateral discussions. Even as the US security alliance forms a vital component of the Indo-Pacific's security architecture, Australia, India and Japan, have pursued closer strategic ties testifying to the evolving strategic glue driving minilateralism across the Indo-Pacific. Although security has been a key driver of such initiatives, countries are discussing how to cooperate on other urgent transnational issues like the pandemic, climate change, cybersecurity and supply chain resilience (Madan, 2021).

Economic Minilateralism

Conversely, India's reticence toward non-security minilaterals, that cover issues like trade, health, digital and technology issues, stems from its economic position and incoherent foreign economic policy that has yet to sift between and reconcile tensions between development interests representing trade and agriculture and industrial interests that are forming around digital services industries. For decades, India's interests have aligned with developing countries in the international order; in practice, this alignment meant caucusing with other developing countries at UN fora to protect Indian interests and project common positions versus developed countries who generally had different interests and priorities on issues like trade and climate change (Nachiappan, 2020). Yet, this reality has largely passed. Minilateral discussions have come to complement and, occasionally, function as a substitute for traditional multilateral discussions. These formal organizations are increasingly being trumped by an astonishing array of flexible groupings whose focus, membership, and activities rest on contingent interests, shared values and incumbent resolve. In recent years, we have witnessed a steady rise in minilateral and plurilateral groups and initiatives spanning functional areas like trade, technology, security and climate change (Naim, 2009).

China's rise and China-US tensions have also influenced the rise and relevance of minilateral frameworks covering economic issues. Since the Obama years and more so under Trump, American officials have sought to arrest China's economic ascent by either establishing alternate fora where US allies and partners discuss rules covering global economic issues or diplomatically restraining China through UN agencies having realized that China relies on the multilateral system for its economic success (Bown and Kolb, 2021). The latter approach raises costs for China since the legitimacy of the Chinese Communist Party emanates from sustaining economic growth which makes Beijing cognizant of and sensitive to concerns regarding its foreign economic policies. Alongside the raft of economic sanctions and tariffs that Washington levied on Beijing from 2018, the Trump administration has also sought to use minilateral frameworks to sideline China on technology issues like 5G and artificial intelligence (AI).

The Trump administration's technological onslaught against Beijing has ushered a slew of efforts to decouple American allies and partners from China's technological ecosystem and key firms like Huawei (Swanson and McCabe, 2020). US efforts to protect 5G technologies and shield it from Chinese control have precipitated multilateral discussions between American allies and partners in Europe and Asia through the Prague 5G Security Conference (Lowell, 2021). The objective of the Prague conference and discussions was to devise proposals to protect countries and firms from growing cyber threats, particularly those related to questionable 'suppliers' like Huawei, and strengthen domestic legal architectures from their activities (Kewalramani, 2020). Globally, G7 countries and select partners have discussed global rules covering AI, largely through the scope of ethics at the Global Partnership on AI (GPAI). The forum was created to devise norms that can regulate how countries develop AI tools and deploy them given prevailing fears around how China and Russia were openly deploying AI tools to undermine civil liberties. GPAI (originally called the International Panel on Artificial Intelligence) was established to address ethical questions and issues around AI, devise rules and principles that would guide AI development in specific countries (Hamidouche, 2021). Michael Kratsios, White House's chief technology officer, hoped that the GPAI could serve as an important "check on China's approach to AI" given China's efforts to deploy AI and other digital tools to manage public safety and order during the pandemic (O'Brien, 2020).

Unlike security issues, India has not openly participated and sought to shape rules and norms on such emergent economic issues at various minilateral frameworks. Participation has been contingent on how these rule and norm making processes affect domestic economic interests, despite calls to support G7 partners on such issues to address China's dominance. So far, India has remained passive on multilateral discussions covering 5G technologies at the Prague Conference while leaving the door open, until recent tensions with China, for Huawei's participation in India's 5G network (Kewalramani, 2020). The Prague conference framework will likely expand these discussions focusing on shared best practices and tools to tackle emergent 5G security threats. These discussions will be important for New Delhi given ongoing issues related to 5G development and the inclusion of Huawei as a domestic operator (Chikermane, 2021). Likewise, although India is a GPAI member, it has largely emphasized the business and development case of AI without wading into the ethical implications, which are of immense importance to domestic governance, given ongoing questions around the erosion of constitutional rights by the current government (Marda, 2020).

On trade, frameworks like the TPP, Transatlantic Trade and Investment Partnership, and the Regional Comprehensive Economic Cooperation Agreement (RCEP) have discussed how to draft new rules to govern cross border trade, including emergent digital issues like e-commerce, data sharing and transfer (Cook and Hoang, 2020; Desierto, 2017). As the ability of the World Trade Organization (WTO) to negotiate emergent trade issues has waned, these competing minilateral frameworks have assumed greater importance with countries looking to use such vehicles to remove existing digital trade barriers. These digital barriers have become vital given the prevalence of digital applications and services during the Covid-19 pandemic. Countries, more than before, are looking to use various rules and laws under the guise of 'data localization' to regulate their digital industries with implications for cross border trade. Such rules have become more common given the inability of the WTO to negotiate digital trade multilaterally; localization decrees generally favour domestic over foreign technology firms given the nature of obligations, particularly when it comes to data, that foreign firms must follow (Basu, 2020). Although WTO rules can potentially resolve these matters under the rubric of digital trade, including data, the desire to move along these lines has not been forthcoming given political difficulties and little appetite from key countries like the United States and China and the EU (Hodson, 2019). With the Doha Round on life support, multilateral rule-making on digital issues has shifted from the WTO to other avenues— bilateral, regional, and plurilateral. Digital trade matters are being negotiated through several plurilateral trade agreements including the Comprehensive and Progressive Agreement for Trans-Pacific Partnership and RCEP.

India has rejected plurilateral trade frameworks, especially RCEP, that cover a range of economic issues like data and labor under trade. In 2012 RCEP negotiations commenced, seeking to cover "goods, services, investments, economic and technical cooperation, competition and intellectual property rights" (Wignaraja, 2013). Countries negotiating the RCEP, including India, hoped to reduce or completely remove all tariff and non-tariff barriers on imports and exports. Indian trade officials were aware of India's shaky trade balance and competitiveness—and that, for various reasons, India had a trade deficit with most RCEP countries including several ASEAN countries, South Korea, China and Australia that remained north of $100 billion in 2019 (Pant, 2019). Given India's waning competitiveness in industries, like dairy and manufacturing, firms in these sectors would have found it difficult to export commodities to Asian markets. Deteriorating export potentials constrained pleas for greater market access; if anything, firms in these industries would have ostensibly compelled Indian trade negotiators to desist from conceding greater access to the Indian market.

Service gains through RCEP for India could have nudged Indian negotiators to accept short term losses through the progressive entry of goods from RCEP countries into the Indian market. Trade agreements like RCEP are generally compromises, where countries exchange market access in areas where they have competitive advantages - in India's case this was clearly services where a trade surplus existed with most ASEAN countries. But RCEP did not move the needle here for India; concessions offered by other countries in terms of accepting Indian professionals, specifically from the IT and software industry, were negligible (Gaur, 2020). Neither was Delhi moved by liberal interpretations of regulating data within RCEP negotiations, signalling its preference for national control in this area, which was largely opposed by other RCEP countries (Nachiappan, 2019). In fact, Indian officials were worried that signing could potentially entrench the market dominance of foreign technology companies without any recourse to small and medium sized technology companies in the Indian market that require sustained access to data to fuel their growth. India has consistently pushed for global data rules that advance the role of the Indian state. This tack was front and centre at the 2019 Osaka G20 Summit, where India opposed the Osaka Track that called for data sharing between leading economies (Basu, 2021). Unsurprisingly, India's positions have been an extension of their domestic policy ambitions, embracing 'data sovereignty', countering 'data colonialism' and retaining publicly generated data to propel state power, particularly when it comes to public service delivery and welfare provision (Joshi, 2020).

Despite disagreements on norms governing development and deployment of emerging technologies, Indian officials, alongside Japanese and Australian counterparts, have found common ground on fortifying supply chains, launching the Resilient Supply Chain Initiative (RSCI) 'to reduce long-term exclusive reliance on Chinese products and technology' (Scott, 2021). It appears security implications, particularly India's trade dependence vis-a-vis China, has spurred Delhi's embrace of the RSCI, which seeks to overcome China's dominance of production networks and supply chains by incentivizing firms to relocate production. Thus, far, Japan, India and Australia are supporting efforts to reroute production networks away from China given Covid-19 supply shocks. India's interest also stems from its potential as a venue for long term manufacturing, particularly goods currently produced in China. Both Japan and India (and the United States through the Quad) are helping finance the production of goods like vaccines in India (Madan, 2021). The necessity to relocate production from China triggers new opportunities for countries like India but the efficacy of minilateral initiatives will likely hinge on the domestic organization of labour and capital to spur output.

Covid-19 has elevated such narrower, more targeted forms of multilateralism. Some minilateral mechanisms will likely proliferate, becoming a staple of international politics despite limited evidence that these frameworks are more effective or yield intended gains for participating states (Patrick, 2020). While these minilateral forums appear amenable to create, run and use to address specific policy problems like maritime security or pandemics, they lack institutional depth; most mechanisms struggle to hold states accountable and uphold avowed commitments. Accountability appears non-existent. Outcomes or the public goods generated are likely to be narrow with gains accruing to a few states at the expense of broader objectives that only more formalized regimes and international organizations pursue (Tan, 2020). Doubts also exist on whether and how these initiatives can contribute and feed into formal multilateral activities, particularly discussions convened by mainstream international organizations, and whether they can foster conducive talks that could redound to shape durable international rules and norms.

Moreover, risks exist for developing countries like India that have long caucused with other developing countries at traditional international organizations to press their interests and claims (Mohan, 2010). Organizations under the UN umbrella, where groupings like the G-77 operate, have given India and other developing countries security and protections when negotiating rules to tackle challenges like climate change, trade and disarmament against developed countries whose interests generally differ (Efstathopoulos and Kelly, 2014). Under UN frameworks, it is difficult to impose or coerce developing countries to accept rules that undermine their interests; in addition, developing countries also invariably use this remit, afforded by international organizations, to introduce alternative or counter hegemonic discourses, like the Common but Differentiated Responsibilities discourse to mitigate global warming, to manage collective action issues the best they see fit (Dubash, 2013). Thus, the introduction and proliferation of narrow coalition-based minilaterals (and plurilaterals) renders such strategies inapplicable for developing countries, testing their resolve and approach while negotiating multilateral matters with developed countries. Increasingly, agendas could be set by a specific set of priorities to achieve concomitant outcomes that require minimal deliberation and quick action.

Minilaterals, however, compel Indian officials to clarify and rethink their economic interests given their narrow nature, specific purpose, loose organization and penchant to prioritize speed over deliberation. Agreements like the TPP, RCEP, and a litany of technology-oriented frameworks like the Prague Conference, GPAI, and Mission Technology Control Regime, and security frameworks like the Quad could potentially harm India's overall economic interests just as they advance geopolitical objectives, specifically aligning and collaborating with 'like-minded' partners like the United States, Japan and other democracies to counter China's rise. India's diffident and defensive response to these minilateral economic frameworks before and post-Covid-19 outbreak suggest reservations exist in New Delhi when committing to rules and agreements that undermine India's development agenda and interests.

India's withdrawal from the RCEP, more than other agreements or negotiations, attests to this unease. However, for India to openly engage and benefit from such minilateral economic initiatives, New Delhi must further align its economic policies with that of key partners like the United States, Australia, Japan and the European Union. Covid-19 has turbocharged India's digitalization which has made these interests ascendant relative to other industrial interests. How the current and future Indian governments negotiate this domestic tussle will likely determine India's appetite toward economic minilateralism.

WHO, the Gates Foundation and Vaccine Multilateralism

As Covid-19 spread, it fell to the WHO to organize a multilateral response. The WHO's role in a crisis like Covid-19 is to provide technical assistance and emergency support to member states exposed and function as a catalyst for coordinating financial resources and personnel to countries most affected. But the WHO's ability to discharge these functions was constrained by two incumbent challenges. First is the WHO's chronic underfunding over the past decade and the rise of new philanthropic actors, especially the Gates Foundation that has become a major force funding global health campaigns jointly with WHO officials and independently on issues like polio, HIV/AIDS, and malaria (Harman, 2016).[1] The second is an immediate constraint—the ongoing geopolitical tussle between China and the United States (Huang, 2020a).

The WHO's coronavirus response was lambasted by critics who felt the organization had been too cozy with the Chinese regime. Few critics, however, noted the WHO's predicament—it had to yield to get the requisite information from Chinese officials to mount a viable response; publicly chastising China, as the WHO did during the SARS epidemic in 2003, could have shut their access to the country potentially increasing global vulnerabilities (Huang, 2020a; Bollyky and Huang, 2021). Simply put, the WHO has transformed structurally and institutionally, which has reduced its capability to act decisively, allowing other actors to step in and fill the vacuum.

With WHO constrained financially and politically and China and the US squabbling over the WHO's role in handling the pandemic, the multilateral effort to tackle Covid-19 was led by a new coalition—France and Germany—which picked up the mantle with the International Monetary Fund, the influential Gates Foundation and its offshoots, Global Alliance for Vaccination and Immunization (GAVI) and the Global Fund (Al Jazeera, 2020). Combined, these forces, governmental, non-governmental and transnational, led the multilateral response around diagnostics, therapeutics and vaccines for Covid-19 by deploying capital and establishing scientific efforts that could produce diagnostic breakthroughs and distribute them globally. With GAVI's support, WHO also established COVAX, the multilateral facility that would provide developed vaccines for low and middle-income countries (Global Alliance for Vaccination and Immunization, 2020).[2] GAVI enlisted major vaccine manufacturers like India's Serum Institute to produce approved vaccines, notably the AstraZeneca jab, for global distribution (Goldhill, 2021).

The WHO has, in effect, evolved to function as a convener and information dispenser that could provide global legitimacy to the efforts being spearheaded by philanthropic organisations and transnational partnerships with European support. The World Health Assembly (WHA) acquired greater importance to ensure ongoing transnational efforts around diagnostics and vaccines could be calibrated with national health agendas and priorities as countries like India battled to mitigate Covid-19 (Brilliant et al., 2021). In fact, WHO's importance only increased for developing countries that lacked both vaccines and necessary medical supplies and therapeutics to mobilize immediate responses to break chains of Covid-19 transmission.

As the coronavirus spread in 2020, India could have assisted the WHO support developing countries secure access to Covid-19 drugs, diagnostics and vaccines being developed without constraint. India also became the head of the WHO's Executive Board, another platform through which New Delhi could emphasize and highlight vaccine equity, especially for developing countries as they countered the pandemic (World Health Organization, 2020).[3] Despite its new leadership position at the WHO and decades of experience supporting developing countries through WHO's regional bureau in South and South East Asia, Indian officials appeared slow and flatfooted to push the WHO to ensure vaccines could be universally available and accessible for developing countries, submitting to the Gates

Foundation's vaccine orthodoxy that pushed for vaccine manufacturers to retain intellectual rights over vaccine development and profits thereafter.

India's inclination to shape this ad-hoc multilateral response was constrained by commercial exigencies tied to domestic vaccine production and the compulsion to support Indian pharma companies that have long drawn financial support from the Gates Foundation to produce vaccines. The Gates Foundation's neoliberal agenda, particularly vis-à-vis vaccines, and its clout over the WHO's institutional agenda coupled with its support for vaccine production in India appears to have complicated India's global health responsibilities, specifically whether to politically champion the cause of global vaccine equity. As WHO member states were discussing how to design a multilateral vaccine initiative, the Gates plan that supported pharma companies to 'hold exclusive rights to lifesaving medicines' found sway and was strewn into the WHO's COVAX program that enshrined monopoly patent rights when developing and deploying vaccines worldwide (Mookim, 2021).

Existing commercial and research partnerships between Indian Pharma, especially the Serum Institute of India and Bharat Biotech, and the Gates Foundation hamstrung India's ability to support global vaccine equity. In fact, the Serum Institute, India's largest vaccine producer, has received grants from the Gates Foundation since November 2012 including $150 million in May 2020 to produce 100 million doses of AstraZeneca vaccine for GAVI (Reuters, 2020). Bharat Biotech, the producer of India's indigenous vaccine Covaxin, received $19 million from the Gates Foundation in 2019 (Tarfe, 2021). Before Covaxin, Bharat Biotech was the first Indian pharma company to receive multiple grants from the Gates Foundation to develop new vaccines for Malaria and Rotavirus (Tarfe, 2021). In early 2021 India's Serum Institute signed a commercial agreement with GAVI to provide COVAX with nearly 1 billion doses of Covishield with 100 million doses due in May 2021 (Goldhill, 2021). Although COVAX hoped to secure vaccines from multiple manufacturers, around three-quarters of doses came from the Serum Institute. In this context, Indian officials refrained from pushing for global and domestic pharma companies to share their vaccine technologies and know-how to manufacturers across the Global South; indeed, such a move would have meant sacrificing patent rights and commercial interests of the Serum Institute and Bharat Biotech.

India's diffidence on deprioritizing patent rights globally, particularly through COVAX, was influenced by the reality that India's interests on vaccines and vaccine equity diverged from that of WHO. Private actors have amassed clout in determining the contours of India's vaccine policy and diplomacy. In fact, India became the first country worldwide 'to place the vaccines in the hands of the private sector, at terms favourable to industry' (Krishnan and Nabia, 2021). In March 2021 New Delhi announced it would procure 50% of vaccine stocks from the Serum Institute and Bharat BioTech with remaining stocks earmarked for state governments and private sector providers at market prices (Alluri, 2021). Instead of negotiating a bulk price with both vaccine manufacturers and thereafter purchasing their supplies for domestic and global distribution, the Modi government deferred to the Serum Institute and Bharat BioTech, resulting in prices that constrained vaccine access.

India's vaccine diplomacy initiative (Vaccine Maitri) also possibly nudged India away from advancing equitable vaccine multilateralism through the WHO and COVAX. Soon after Delhi approved Covishield and Covaxin, the government commenced a sprawling effort to export them worldwide, despite concerns raised on whether sufficient domestic supplies existed should a second wave hit (MEA, 2020). Undoubtedly, the vaccine diplomacy campaign grew from India's capability in producing vaccines and generic medicines that other countries relied on; the exercise, however, came out of a wily calculus—the pandemic was ebbing in India in early 2021, and there was enough supply of vaccine doses to share and sharing will enhance India's diplomatic standing in South Asia and beyond.

Indeed, the effort appears to have been driven not only as an opportunity to amass goodwill among neighbours but carve pathways for Indian Covid-19 vaccines in other countries just as China's vaccine diplomacy took shape (Binder and Northrop, 2021). Since early 2021 India has exported 66 million vaccine doses worldwide, primarily to countries in South Asia, the Middle East and Africa (MEA, 2021). Besides the Serum Institute's Covishield Vaccine, the second most-used Covid-19 vaccine worldwide, New Delhi has shipped nearly 20 million Covaxin doses produced by Bharat Biotech (MEA, 2021). Although draped and presented in altruistic tones, India's vaccine diplomacy has largely been a commercial one - of the 66 million doses exported, only 10 million were provided non-commercially (MEA, 2021).

India's transactional relationship with COVAX engendered a scenario where vaccines represented a product that advanced specific interests at the expense of broader global public goods, particularly vaccine access and equity. Initial supporters of COVAX include a range of countries including the US, UK, Canada, Japan, Australia, New Zealand, UAE, France, Germany, Italy, Spain, Sweden, and Portugal (Global Alliance for Vaccination and Immunization, 2021). All these countries pledged money and surplus doses from their supplies for low- and middle-income countries. India was conspicuously silent despite internal efforts to produce several vaccines including the Serum Institute-produced AstraZeneca vaccine. The Indian government's distorted vaccine policy, transactional vaccine diplomacy and disinclination to centre vaccine equity at global health discussions has had ripple effects across other developing countries, especially in South Asia and Africa, that were heavily dependent on Indian vaccines. Nepal halted its domestic vaccination drive after Indian vaccine supplies dried up (Ethirajan, 2021). Some 40 African countries that relied on COVAX and the Serum Institute to obtain their share of jabs were left in the cold (Paruvacini, 2021).

The rise of private actors has transformed global health governance (Rushton and Williams, 2011; Fidler, 2010). These private actors, especially philanthropic foundations like the Gates Foundation and pharmaceutical companies like the Serum Institute, have brought vast resources and capacities to help tackle and address various global health problems (McCoy and McGoey, 2011). In less than two decades, these private actors have injected new ideas, resources and innovations into the global health architecture that have altered the multilateral governance of public health (Dodgson et al., 2017). Covid-19 has increased their importance to both multilateral organizations like the WHO that rely on them for funding and states like India who partner with these actors to produce and deliver various public goods. That said, these actors have their own distinct interests which could clash with and undermine the priorities of multilateral organizations and states (Clinton and Sridhar, 2017). The political clout of the Gates Foundation in global health and capabilities of the Serum Institute vis-à-vis vaccination has complicated the equitable provision of vaccines worldwide with limited recourse for those at their whim or looking to check their power.

Conclusion

This chapter has covered how India has responded to two institutional shifts in global governance that Covid-19 has accelerated - the rise of minilateralism and influential non-state actors like the Gates Foundation that work with states to mobilize multilateral coalitions to tackle trans-boundary challenges like Covid-19. Multilateralism is being buffeted by geopolitical exigencies, specifically US-Chinese tensions, and structural considerations related to capacity, financing and operational constraints that has seen the proliferation of minilateral policymaking and the rise of non-state actors like the Gates Foundation play important multilateral roles. Increasing operational and financial constraints at multilateral organizations at the backdrop of great power tensions, that Covid-19 has only intensified and exacerbated, has not only pushed minilaterals to the fore but also affected the basis of multilateral action and coordination with various non-state actors engaged.

India has responded tepidly to economic minilateral initiatives, particularly those covering trade, technologies and digital issues while contributing robustly to security-focused minilaterals like the Quad and related maritime security initiatives. Unsure of how to commit to new forms of economic minilateralism given domestic economic transitions, India has remained cautious and distant, opting to let other countries discuss and decide how to devise rules and commitments to integrate their economies, particularly on digital issues. In contrast, India's eagerness to deploy domestically manufactured vaccines through bilateral means has complicated and constrained its multilateral obligations to WHO, specifically vaccine equity. Economic considerations, specifically commercial interests of Indian vaccine manufacturers like the Serum Institute and Bharat BioTech, and the ties both companies have cultivated with the Gates Foundation, have cooled India's attitudes toward advancing global vaccine equity.

Going ahead, India should assess how these new patterns of multilateralism and new actors driving and constraining genuine multilateral campaigns align with and affect its economic, political and security interests. Indian officials must become more agile in shaping emergent standards and rules to ensure domestic firms can access foreign markets and balancing those particular economic interests with that of supporting the provision of global public goods like vaccines that enhance India's diplomatic heft. The trade-offs are fine and the implications immense. A reticent India when it comes to adjusting to these shifts in global governance could likely mean losing space in shaping future rules governing vital economic areas like digital trade, including the adoption of standards and rules that reflect the interests of other countries, chiefly the United States or China, compelling India to either accede to or reject such rules.

Notes

1 Although the World Health Organization is managed by member states which donate funds, it increasingly relies on private donors to function. The biggest donor is the Gates Foundation, the largest private contributor to the WHO, providing roughly 10% of its budget.
2 COVAX brings together governments, global health organizations, manufacturers, scientists, private sector, civil society and philanthropy, with the aim of providing innovative and equitable access to Covid-19 diagnostics, treatments and vaccines to end the pandemic. The focus of COVAX is to ensure that people in all corners of the world will get access to Covid-19 vaccines once they are available, regardless of their wealth. (WHO, 2020)
3 The World Health Assembly (WHA) is the WHO's main decision-making body made up of 194 Member States. The WHO Board and the Assembly create a forum where debate occurs on health issues and for addressing concerns raised by WHO member states. Both the WHO Board and the WHA produce three kinds of documents — resolutions passed, official WHO publications, and other official documents.

References

Al Jazeera. "Coronavirus research gets $500 million in pledges at Paris Forum, November 12, 2020. www.aljazeera.com/economy/2020/11/12/coronavirus-resea rch-gets-500m-in-pledges-at-paris-forum.

Alluri, Aparna. *"India's Covid vaccine shortage: The desperate wait gets longer,"* BBC News, May 1, 2021. www.bbc.com/news/world-asia-india-56912977.

Anuar, Amalina and Nazia Hussain. *Minilateralism for Multilateralism in the Post-Covid Age.* S. Rajaratnam School of International Studies. http://hdl.handle.net/11540/13108. (2021).

Basu, Arindrajit. "The Retreat of the Data Localization Brigade: India, Indonesia and Vietnam." *The Diplomat*, no. 10. https://thediplomat.com/2020/01/the-retreat-of-th e-data-localization-brigade-india-indonesia-and-vietnam. (2020).

Basu, Arindrajit. "Sovereignty in a 'datafied' world: A framework for Indian diplomacy." ORF Digital Frontiers, Observer Research Foundation, May 2, 2021. www.orfonline.org/expert-speak/sovereignty-datafied-world-framework-indian-diplomacy.

Binder, Eli and Katrina Northrop. "Shots in the Dark." The Wire China, May 5, 2021. www.thewirechina.com/2021/05/02/shots-in-the-dark.

Bollyky, Thomas and Yanzhong Huang. "The Right Way to Investigate the Origins of COVID-19." *Foreign Affairs*, August 2021. www.foreignaffairs.com/articles/china/2021-08-12/right-way-investigate-origins-covid-19.

Bown, Chad and Melina Kolb. "Trump's Trade War Timeline: An Up-to-Date Guide." Trade and Investment Policy Watch, Peterson Institute for International Economics. October 4, 2021. www.piie.com/blogs/trade-investment-policy-watch/trump-trade-war-china-date-guide.

Brilliant et al. "The Forever Virus A Strategy for the Long Fight Against COVID-19." *Foreign Affairs*, July/August 2021.

Chikermane, Gautam. "5G Infrastructure, Huawei's Techno-Economic Advantages and India's National Security Concerns: An Analysis." *ORF Occasional Paper*, no. 226 (2019): 62.

Clinton, Chelsea and Devi Sridhar. *Governing Global Health: who runs the world and why?*. Oxford University Press, 2017.

Cook, Malcolm and Hoang Thi Ha. "Beyond China, the USA and ASEAN: Informal Minilateral Options." *ISEAS Perspectives*, no. 63 (2020): 1–9.

Desierto, Diane A. "ASEAN Investment Treaties, RCEP, and CPTPP: Regional Strategies, Norms, Institutions, and Politics." *Wash. Int'l LJ*, no. 27 (2017): 349.

Dodgson, Richard, Kelley Lee, and Nick Drager. *Global Health Governance, a conceptual review*. Routledge, 2017.

Dubash, N.K. "The politics of climate change in India: narratives of equity and co-benefits." *Wiley Interdisciplinary Reviews: Climate Change*, 4, no. 3 (2013.): 191–201.

Efstathopoulos, Charalampos and Dominic Kelly. "India, developmental multilateralism and the Doha ministerial conference." *Third World Quarterly*, 35, no. 6 (2014): 1066–1081.

Ethirajan, Anbarasan. "As India halts vaccine exports, Nepal faces its own Covid crisis." BBC News, May 12, 2021. www.bbc.com/news/world-asia-57055209.

Fidler, David P. "The challenges of global health governance." Council on Foreign Relations, 2010.

Global Alliance for Vaccination and Immunization. "World leaders unite to commit to global equitable access for COVID-19 vaccines." June 2, 2021. www.gavi.org/news/media-room/world-leaders-unite-commit-global-equitable-access-covid-19-vaccines.

Goldhill, Olivia. 'Naively ambitious': How COVAX failed on its promise to vaccinate the world: Special Report.' October 8, 2021. www.statnews.com/2021/10/08/how-covax-failed-on-its-promise-to-vaccinate-the-world.

Hamidouche, Karim. "Artificial Intelligence: A New Tool for Diplomats." In *Artificial Intelligence and Digital Diplomacy*. Cham: Springer, 2021: pp. 25–32.

Harman, Sophie. "The Bill and Melinda Gates Foundation and legitimacy in global health governance." *Global Governance* (2016): 349–368.

Haruko, Wada. The Indo-Pacific Concept: Geographical Adjustments and their Implications. RSIS Working Paper, Nanyang Technological University, www.rsis.edu.sg/wp-content/uploads/2020/03/WP326.pdf.

Hodson, Susannah. "Applying WTO and FTA disciplines to data localization measures." *World Trade Review*, 18, no. 4 (2019): 579–607.

Hopewell, Kristen. "Recalcitrant spoiler? Contesting dominant accounts of India's role in global trade governance." *Third World Quarterly*, 39, no. 3 (2018): 577–593.

Huang, Yanzhong. *"How coronavirus is poisoning US-China relations, one accusation at a time."* *South China Morning Post*, June 17, 2020. www.scmp.com/comment/opinion/a rticle/3089131/how-coronavirus-poisoning-us-china-relations-one-accusation-time.

Huang, Yanzhong. "China's Public Health Response to the COVID-19 Outbreak." *China Leadership Monitor*, June 2020. www.prcleader.org/huang.

Hurrell, Andrew and Amrita Narlikar. "A new politics of confrontation? Brazil and India in multilateral trade negotiations." *Global Society*, 20, no. 4 (2006): 415–433.

Johnston, Lauren A. "The Belt and Road Initiative: what is in it for China?." *Asia & the Pacific Policy Studies*, 6, no. 1 (2019): 40–58.

Joshi, Divij. "Interrogating India's quest for data sovereignty." *Seminar*, July 2020, www.india-seminar.com/2020/731/731_divij_joshi.htm.

Kewalramani, Manoj. "Going slow on 5G: India's approach." *Seminar*, July 2020, www.india-seminar.com/2020/731/731_manoj_kewalramani.htm.

Krishnan, Vidya and Sarah Nabia. "The Indian government used the pandemic to craft a political image and failed to save lives." *Caravan India*, September 14, 2021. https://caravanmagazine.in/health/the-indian-government-used-the-pandemic-to-cra ft-a-political-image.

Le Thu, Huong. "The Quadrilateral Security Dialogue and ASEAN centrality." In *Minilateralism in the Indo-Pacific*. Abingdon: Routledge, 2020: pp. 88–102.

Lowell, Kirsten S. "The New" Arms" Race: How the US and China Are Using Government Authorities in the Race to Control 5G Wearable Technology." *Geo. Mason Int'l LJ*, 12 (2021): 1.

Madan, Tanvi. "More than hype: Summit shows that the Quad is already coming of age." *The Times of India*, September 25, 2021. https://timesofindia.indiatimes.com/ blogs/voices/more-than-hype-summit-shows-that-the-quad-is-already-coming-of-age.

Marda, Vidushi. "India and global artificial intelligence governance." *Seminar*, July 2020, www.india-seminar.com/2020/731/731_vidushi_marda.htm.

Mitchell et al. "China and Covid-19: what went wrong in Wuhan?." *Financial Times*, October 18, 2020, www.ft.com/content/82574e3d-1633-48ad-8afb-71ebb3fe3dee.

Ministry of External Affairs, Government of India. *"Vaccine Maitri."* September 14, 2021, www.mea.gov.in/vaccine-supply.htm.

Mohan, C. Raja. "Rising India: partner in shaping the global commons?." *The Washington Quarterly*, 33, no. 3 (2010): 133–148.

Mohan, C Raja. "The Changing Dynamics of India's Multilateralism." In Sidhu, Waheguru PalSingh, PratapBhanu Mehta, and Bruce D. Jones, eds. *Shaping the emerging world: India and the multilateral order*. Washington, DC: Brookings Institution Press, 2013.

Mookim, Mohit. *"The World Loses Under Bill Gates' Vaccine Colonialism."* *The Wired Magazine*, May 19, 2021, www.wired.com/story/opinion-the-world-lose s-under-bill-gates-vaccine-colonialism.

Nachiappan, Karthik. *Does India Negotiate?*. Oxford: Oxford University Press, 2020.

Naim, Moises. "Minilateralism." *Foreign Policy*, June 21, 2009, https://foreignpolicy. com/2009/06/21/minilateralism.

O'Brien, Matt. "US joins G7 artificial intelligence group to counter China." *AP News*, May 29, 2020, https://apnews.com/article/682cbe41b96d32bc4cf5b6ec42853a69.

Pant, Harsh. "Modi Was Right. India Isn't Ready for Free Trade." *Foreign Policy*, November 19, 2019. https://foreignpolicy.com/2019/11/19/modi-pull-out-rcep-india -manufacturers-compete-china.

Paruvacini, Giulia. "India's halt to vaccine exports 'very problematic' for Africa." Reuters, May 16, 2021, www.reuters.com/business/healthcare-pharmaceuticals/indias-halt-vaccine-exports-very-problematic-africa-2021-05-18.

Patrick, Stewart. "The New "New Multilateralism": Minilateral Cooperation, but at What Cost?." *Global Summitry*, 1, no. 2 (2015): 115–134.

Patrick, Stewart. "When the system fails." *Foreign Affairs*, 99 (2020): 40.

Piccone, Ted. "UN Human Rights Council: As the US returns, it will have to deal with China and its friends." *Order from Chaos*, Brookings Institution, February 25, 2021, www.brookings.edu/blog/order-from-chaos/2021/02/25/un-human-rights-council-as-the-us-returns-it-will-have-to-deal-with-china-and-its-friends.

Rajagopalan, Rajeshwari Pillai. "Explaining the Rise of Minilaterals in the Indo-Pacific." ORF Special Report, September 16, 2021. www.orfonline.org/research/explaining-the-rise-of-minilaterals-in-the-indo-pacific.

Reuters. "India's Serum Institute to get $150 million from Gates Foundation for COVID-19 vaccine." August 7, 2020, www.reuters.com/article/us-health-coronavirus-india-vaccine-idUSKCN2531B4.

Roy, Vikram. *"Indian drug firm joins Gates Foundation in drive to provide cheap Covid vaccine."* RFI News, September 8, 2020, www.rfi.fr/en/asia/20200809-indian-drug-firm-joins-gates-foundation-in-drive-to-provide-cheap-covid-vaccine.

Rushton, Simon and Owain Williams, eds. *Partnerships and foundations in global health governance*. Cham: Springer, 2011.

Scott, J. "Australia, Japan and India Form Supply Chain Initiative to Counter China." Bloomberg, April 28, 2021. www.bloombergquint.com/global-economics/supply-chain-initiative-from-japan-india-australia-under-way.

Singh, Bhubhindar and Sarah Teo. "Introduction: Minilateralism in the Indo-Pacific." In *Minilateralism in the Indo-Pacific*. Abingdon: Routledge, 2020: pp. 1–12.

Singh, Teshu. "China and the Air Defense Identification Zone." Institute of Peace and Conflict Studies, www.files.ethz.ch/isn/176944/SR148-IPCSSpecialFocus-ADIZ.pdf.

Swanson, A. and McCabe, D., 2020. "Trump's effort to keep US tech out of China alarms American Firms." *The New York Times*, February 17, 2020: 16.

Tan, See Seng. "ASEAN Defence Ministers' Meeting-Plus: Multilateralism mimicking minilateralism?." In *Minilateralism in the Indo-Pacific*. Abingdon: Routledge, 2020: pp. 120–134.

Tarfe, Akshay. "Why Are Indians So Angry at Bill Gates?." *The Diplomat*, June 15, 2021. https://thediplomat.com/2021/06/why-are-indians-so-angry-at-bill-gates.

Tillett, Andrew and Emma Connors. "New bloc of Australia, India, Indonesia takes shape amid China fears." *Australian Financial Review*, September 4, 2020, www.afr.com/politics/federal/new-bloc-of-australia-india-indonesia-takes-shape-amid-china-fears-20200904-p55sec.

Tirkey, Aarshi. "Minilateralism: Weighing the Prospects for Cooperation and Governance." *ORF Issue Brief*, No. 489, September 2021, Observer Research Foundation.

Tow, William T. "Minilateralism and US security policy in the Indo-Pacific: The legacy, viability and deficiencies of a new security approach." In *Minilateralism in the Indo-Pacific*. Abingdon: Routledge, 2020: pp. 13–26

Wignarajah, Ganeshan. "Why the RCEP matters for Asia and the world." East Asia Forum, May 15, 2013, www.eastasiaforum.org/2013/05/15/why-the-rcep-matters-for-asia-and-the-world.

Woods, Ngaire. "Good Governance in International Organizations." In *Understanding Global Cooperation*. Brill, 2021. pp. 92–115

World Health Organization. "India elected chair of WHO's Executive Board." News Reports Division, SEARO, May 22, 2020, www.who.int/southeastasia/news/detail/22-05-2020-india-elected-chair-of-who-s-executive-board.

World Health Organization. "Report of the WHO-China Joint Mission on Coronavirus Disease 2019(COVID-19)." September 12, 2020, www.who.int/docs/default-source/coronaviruse/who-china-joint-mission-on-covid-19-final-report.pdf.

10 Wasted Opportunity

Covid-19 and Regional Cooperation in South Asia

Surupa Gupta

As a region, South Asia has a reputation of being the least integrated. It is also a region marked by one of the highest rates of multidimensional poverty.[1] At the same time, the South Asian region has been making enormous strides in poverty reduction during the last decade: Bangladesh, India and Nepal were among sixteen countries that were in the forefront of reducing multidimensional poverty. It is also home to some of the fastest growing economies, namely Bangladesh and India. The Covid-19 pandemic stopped such progress in its tracks: poverty rates soared as a result of lockdowns and disruptions in value chains and economic growth rates plummeted. The spread of the pandemic also led countries to re-examine China's role and their dependence on China.

Against such a backdrop, Indian Prime Minister Narendra Modi's initiative of getting South Asian heads of state gathered in a virtual meeting sent a strong message about the need for cooperation. Crises are known to prompt systemic changes at the domestic, regional and international levels. This chapter seeks to assess the impact of the pandemic on cooperation within the region. Did the economic and political fall-out of the pandemic act as a driver for cooperation at the regional and sub-regional levels? Did the states realize the potential for cooperation in the region?

It is important, at the outset, to spell out what this chapter addresses and what it does not. First, the chapter focuses on the region known as South Asia, consisting of the following countries: Afghanistan, Bangladesh, Bhutan, India, Maldives, Nepal, Pakistan, and Sri Lanka. Second, the chapter focuses on two aspects of regional cooperation: economic integration among the countries of the region and cooperation on addressing the impact of the Covid-19 pandemic. Economists have argued for a long time that the region would benefit from economic integration. However, politics has come in the way time and again, leading some of the countries in the region to look for alternative sub-regional groupings. Cooperation, particularly in restoring connectivity in the region, has been growing in recent years.[2] Economic growth—not necessarily an outcome of regional cooperation in this case— has been raising incomes and pulling citizens out of poverty and bringing into focus even more starkly what faster growth the region can achieve if the

DOI: 10.4324/9781003248149-10

barriers to trade and cross-border integration were lifted and if there were easier flow of goods, services and people within the region.

The arrival of the pandemic at such a moment did two things: it reversed decades of progress the region had made in bringing down poverty and provided an opportunity to the smaller countries in the region to rethink their foreign policy choices. It also provided an opportunity for India to restart economic cooperation in the region. In the following section, the chapter discusses the existing literature on the relative successes and failures in cooperation in the region. Next, the chapter provides a brief history of regional cooperation efforts in South Asia. It then describes the economic impact of the pandemic on the region as a whole and on specific countries. In the subsequent section, the chapter outlines the efforts that the region, in general, and India, in particular, made to address the Covid-19 challenge using regional and bilateral frameworks. The chapter then highlights the role China played in the region during the pandemic. It concludes with observations and lessons that emerge out of this discussion.

The trajectory of cooperation in the region had been gradually evolving for a number of years. The geographic focus of integration has shifted to smaller groupings of countries in the region. The issue focus has shifted to building physical infrastructure rather than only pursuing economic integration through cross-border trade and investment.[3] The onset of the pandemic provided the countries in the region both an opportunity and a cause for a reset and for India, another chance to demonstrate its leadership. This chapter argues that the pandemic drove home the fragility of growth and the challenges facing economic cooperation in the region.

As the impact of the pandemic has unfolded, observers have warned of fiscal stress for years to come. Relatedly, economic development challenges complicate the geo-strategic calculus of both India and its neighbors. One aspect of that challenge is that India is both an emerging and fast-growing economy and at the same time, a country with substantial development challenges of its own, which limit its ability to provide public goods for the region. A second challenge arises from the complicated strategic environment: regional cooperation in South Asia has always suffered as a result of the Indo-Pakistani rivalry. Moreover, the entry of China, its increasingly closer relations with Pakistan and its ability and interest in addressing some of the development needs of India's immediate neighbors has created conditions for competition for dominance between India and China. The challenges unleashed by the pandemic created opportunities for both; however, the Indian government's catastrophic handling of the second wave of the pandemic in April-May 2021 and the resultant moratorium on vaccine exports partially undid the goodwill India had earned in the immediate aftermath of Covid-19 outbreak. For regional cooperation in South Asia to advance to the next level, India needs to build its capacity to provide public goods such as vaccines, investment and infrastructure funding so that it can offer an alternative to China's attractiveness as the region's development partner. Some initial success in doing so and in developing issue-based cooperation in building connectivity will likely decrease the incentive for neighbors to engage in cooperative arrangements with China.

Regional Cooperation in South Asia: History and Evolution

South Asia took a step towards a formal mechanism for regional cooperation by setting up the South Asian Association for Regional Cooperation (SAARC) in December 1985. However, regional cooperation has had a shaky start from the very beginning. When Zia-ur Rehman, the late President of Bangladesh proposed creating SAARC, the initial response from India was lukewarm.[4] At the time, India's relations with both Bangladesh and Pakistan faced several challenges. The Indian foreign policy establishment was wary that such an organization would be a place where the smaller countries in the region could "gang-up" against India.[5] At the same time, there were voices that highlighted that integration could be perceived as an opportunity for fostering political stability and economic development. The voices in favor of joining prevailed and SAARC came into existence at its first summit in Dhaka in 1985, with a primary focus on promoting welfare in the region and improving the quality of life of citizens through economic growth and social progress.[6]

When SAARC was established, the security environment was very different from what it is today. India and Pakistan had been locked in an enduring rivalry since their independence from Britain in 1947. By the 1980s the two had fought three wars and had engaged in a race to develop nuclear weapons. While Pakistan and China had started to get closer, China's material power was nowhere near what it is today. India's relations with Bangladesh was entering a difficult phase with border and water-sharing issues as well as Bangladesh's domestic politics complicating their bilateral ties. Sri Lanka was facing a civil war and resented India's rather inept effort to address the threat. The situation is quite different today. While India and Pakistan's rivalry endures and both have acquired nuclear weapons capability, India's 1991 economic reforms and subsequent rethinking on foreign policy has put it on a different and higher growth trajectory. Since the early 1990s, India's integration with the global economy has grown as has its stature in global governance. Among its neighbors, India has been able to improve relations with Bangladesh and Sri Lanka. On the flip side, Pakistan and China have grown closer, most recently with China building the China-Pakistan Economic Corridor and establishing a substantial presence in that country. China has emerged as the largest economy in the world in purchasing power parity terms and during the last decade, under its Belt and Road Initiative, China has provided infrastructure funding to several countries in South Asia.

These changes have created both challenges and opportunities. On the one hand, it has become amply clear that a conventional path to regional cooperation cannot be pursued in South Asia, given Pakistan's role in sponsoring terrorist attacks against India and refusing to offer India trade reciprocity in the form of most favored nation treatment in regional and bilateral trade. On the other, starting with the adoption of the Gujral Doctrine in 1996, India has made much progress towards building a regional framework in which it does not seek reciprocity from its smaller neighbors, such as Bangladesh, Bhutan, Maldives, Nepal, and Sri Lanka, in trade and in other issue areas.[7] As Pakistan's actions have thwarted progress in regional cooperation, India has taken the initiative of building sub-regional groupings such as the Bay of Bengal Initiative for Multisectoral Technical and Economic Cooperation (BIMSTEC) involving India's neighbors to its east and the Bangladesh, Bhutan, India, and Nepal Initiative (BBIN) for improved connectivity among these states. A full discussion of these cooperation efforts is beyond the scope of this chapter. When Narendra Modi became Prime Minister in 2014, his initial focus on a Neighborhood First policy did not yield much by way of positive outcomes. Since 2016 the administration's focus has shifted to BIMSTEC and BBIN, in part because of the challenges of working with Pakistan and in part, because such a focus is essential for building India's relations with east and southeast Asia, which are an integral part of India's Act East and now Indo-Pacific Policy. Efforts at building connectivity in the BIMSTEC region and furthering the BBIN initiative have both been slow processes and the countries have relied on bilateral interaction to strengthen ties and cooperation wherever possible.

Economic Justifications and Political Obstacles

Here we discuss the literature that addresses regional cooperation in South Asia. We focus particularly on the economic dimension of cooperation. Economists have long argued that regional economic integration in South Asia is a sine qua non of economic development in the region. Successful integration will likely also improve security and stability in a region that has seen four wars between India and Pakistan, numerous militant insurgencies and acts of terrorism. While regional integration is not a silver bullet, its positive impact in fostering economic development is well-documented. Regional cooperation is a broader process that focuses on coordinated action on various dimensions including political, strategic, economic, cultural and so on. In South Asia, the effort at regional cooperation began with the establishment of the South Asian Association for Regional Cooperation (SAARC). However, the progress on cooperation, as well as on economic integration has been episodic, fragmented and underwhelming.

The perspective of economists is based mainly on the positive role that cross-border trade purportedly plays in increasing growth rates and decreasing poverty in a region. Even though one of the goals of the SAARC was promoting economic welfare and accelerated economic growth, its initial charge had little to do with economic cooperation.[8] A focus on poverty, operationalized by setting up an independent committee to study it, was the first tangible effort to address economic issues within SAARC. Eventually the member countries agreed to first set up a South Asia Preferential Trade Association in 1995 and subsequently, a South Asian Free Trade Association (SAFTA) was signed in 2004 and ratified in 2006. Intraregional trade has increased modestly over the years but the overall proportion of trade within the region has remained more or less stagnant at 5% since SAFTA came into existence. A recent World Bank report calculates that merchandise trade within the region, which stood at $23 billion in 2015, could potentially have been $67 billion, almost triple that amount, if trade barriers did not exist.[9]

Scholars have ascribed South Asia's modest record in regional cooperation to several factors. Regional economic integration remains limited in part because of SAFTA's design. Two factors limit the growth of trade in the region. First, when SAFTA was negotiated, a large number of goods were added to the sensitive list which includes items that are exempted from trade liberalization—almost 50% of exportable goods from the region were included in the negative list.[10] Second, many countries in the region—particularly Bangladesh, Pakistan, and Sri Lanka—impose para tariffs on their imports.[11] Although not officially recognized as tariffs, para tariffs include regulatory duties, port and airport levies and supplementary levies on imports that their domestic producers do not face. These para tariffs, therefore, act as additional tariffs on imports and inasmuch as they increase protection and decrease transparency, they create an anti-export bias within the region.

Scholars also assign much of the blame for lack of cooperation on the rivalry between India and Pakistan.[12] On various occasions, actions taken by Pakistan in support of terrorist and other activities has led to the postponement of summit meetings.[13] The South Asian Association for Regional Cooperation, for example, has not had a summit meeting since 2014. While the Modi administration's preference for engaging bilaterally might have contributed to this, the terrorist attacks in Uri in 2016 and Pulwama in 2019 have certainly played a key role in India's focus away from SAARC. Following the Uri attack, India invited the heads of state of BIMSTEC to meet on the sidelines of the BRICS meeting in Goa in 2016. Observers interpreted this move as emphasizing the significance and feasibility of BIMSTEC rather than SAARC as the preferred vehicle for regional cooperation.

The effort to revive regional cooperation in the region in the aftermath of the Covid-19 pandemic's outbreak must be seen within this context. In continuation with the trend of combining efforts at regional cooperation with other forms of cooperation, we observe that while a few of the efforts undertaken during the pandemic fit the SAARC framework, much of the provision of public goods such as vaccines and medical supplies has happened under bilateral frameworks that have existed between countries in the region.

The Covid-19 Pandemic and South Asia

In January 2020 news about the spread of a deadly virus emerged from the city of Wuhan in China. A month later, the World Health Organization (WHO) called the spread of the virus a pandemic. Subsequently, in March 2020, most South Asian countries announced lockdown of their economies and most economic activity came to a near halt.

The impact of Covid-19 on South Asia was particularly harsh. After years of falling poverty rates, both the absolute number of poor and the poverty rate increased in almost all the countries. In fact, the World Bank estimated that a majority of those who were impoverished by the pandemic lived in South Asia.[14] Supply chains were interrupted. There were widespread income and job losses. Economic growth rates plunged. Remittances from citizens working in the Middle East, Europe and elsewhere, a major source of income for many countries in the region, temporarily dried up. The region was left with both demand side and supply side challenges. In this section, we focus on the challenges that the South Asian countries faced by examining Covid-19's impact on the five main economies in the region: Bangladesh, India, Nepal, Pakistan, and Sri Lanka.

Covid-19's impact on Bangladesh becomes apparent from evidence from almost all sectors of the economy—manufacturing and services bore the brunt of the pandemic whereas agriculture faced challenges from prolonged floods. Bangladesh has had a remarkable growth story in recent years. Not only did it graduate from a low-income country to a lower middle-income country in 2015, it has sustained an average GDP growth of 7% a year over the past decade.[15] Further, it has shown dramatic success with poverty reduction with the population at the international poverty line falling from 43.5% in 1991 to 14.3% in 2016.[16] With the onset of the pandemic, the government announced a shutdown on March 26, resulting in a slowdown in domestic economic activity. According to World Bank data, GDP growth decelerated from 8.15% in 2019 to 2.38% in 2020. According to a World Bank simulation exercise that took into account the slowdown in GDP growth, the income losses of informal workers and the temporary drop in remittances estimated that the percentage of people below the poverty level had increased to 30%, erasing previous gains; poverty rate was at a comparable level of 31.5% back in 2010 and had been continuously falling since then.[17]

A second source of impact was the slowdown in export of ready-made garments, a sector that makes up over 80% of Bangladesh's overall exports: garment exports fell by 83% year on year in April 2020. One consequence of this was widespread job loss or prolonged absence from work, leading to rising food insecurity. The rural economy, predominantly based on agriculture, also suffered a harsh impact: during the first three months of the pandemic, difficulties included harvest delays, challenges in selling farm produce, input disruptions, and associated cost increases and a decline in non-farm income.

A third source of impact was the fall in remittances – wages sent home by Bangladeshi workers in the Middle East, Britain, the United States and other countries.[18] Between 2010–11 and 2019–20 remittances had risen from $11.6 billion to $18.2 billion, the latter representing almost 6% of the country's GDP in 2019.[19] Based on Bangladesh Bank figures, remittances declined by nearly 24% year on year between April 2019 and April 2020 before gradually recovering from July 2020.[20] Despite initial pessimism, remittances emerged as a bright spot, rising to $24.7 billion in 2020–21.[21] The labor market also showed signs of recovery in early 2021. The country remains dependent on three factors: public expenditure, garment exports and remittances. Its rate of poverty reduction and job creation had declined even before the pandemic hit. Further recovery would be contingent on a successful vaccination effort and in the longer term, on the diversification of products and markets—in all of these areas regional cooperation including integration of markets would be crucial.

As the largest economy in the region, India's vulnerability to and recovery from this pandemic provides substantial insights on the pivotal role of as well as future prospects of cooperation in the region. India had sustained three years of gradually declining GDP growth, registering 4% growth in 2019, before the pandemic hit. A March–May lockdown led to a steep contraction of the economy by 23.9% during April–June 2020 and 7.5% during July–September 2020—these shocks reverberated across various sectors within the economy.[22] The worst hit sectors were manufacturing and services such as construction, all of which employ the more vulnerable sections of the population. The lockdown caused country-wide urban-rural migration of contingent labor. Even though agricultural production was the bright spot in the economy, interruptions in the food supply chain caused high food inflation during the second half of 2020. While India's growth after the first wave of the pandemic and the lifting of the lockdown showed resilience, a subsequent and more deadly second wave caused harm both to the economy and to India's reputation as a major and/or emerging power seeking to play a role in global governance.

Like most South Asian economies, Nepal's experienced growth during 2009–19, even though the average growth rate was more modest, at 4.9%, than Bangladesh's. Nepal's output fell by an estimated 1.9% in 2020.[23] Workers reported that more than two out of every five experienced a loss in job or income in 2020. While remittances, which lifted consumption levels among a large portion of the population during the prior decade, stayed high, job and income losses likely pushed people back into poverty. The lockdown, initiated in response to the pandemic, affected workers in the informal sector and in subsistence activities. A large number of migrant workers returned home. The lockdown also had an adverse impact on tourism and related services, all of which contribute substantially to the economy: tourism makes up 6.7% of Nepal's GDP and employs 6.9% of its workforce.[24] While Nepal was one of the first to receive vaccines from India, continued recovery of the Nepalese economy will depend on continuous supply of vaccines both in the country and in countries that send tourists to it.

Unlike most other economies in South Asia, Pakistan's has been growing more slowly during the last two decades: according to the World Bank, Pakistan's annual per capita growth, at 2%, has remained less than half of the average in the region. The lack of investment and export-fueled growth in the country has repeatedly pushed it to the point where external and fiscal imbalances were unsustainable, forcing the country to access external resources. Most recently, in 2019, Pakistan had to negotiate a 39-month arrangement with the International Monetary Fund's Extended Fund Facility (EFF) to help it tide over the most recent crisis. The pandemic came in the heels of this and led to a 0.5% contraction in Pakistan's GDP. About half the working population experienced job or income loss, with the informal sector taking the biggest hit. The incidence of poverty increased from 4.4% in 2018–19 to 5.4% in 2019–20.[25] The EFF, which supported key macro-economic and sectoral reforms, had to be suspended until 2022. The initial impact was particularly harsh on manufacturing firms in Pakistan: a study recorded that over 90% of all firms faced revenue losses in the initial period of the pandemic.[26]

Robust remittance flows staved off further pain in Pakistan as it did in Bangladesh and in Sri Lanka.[27] The economy is estimated to have performed better in 2020–21, with GDP rising by 3.5%. However, the recovery remains tentative, given challenges such as low vaccination rates, high public debt and the slow pace of much-needed structural reforms. In early 2021 Pakistan indicated that it was reconsidering its decision to halt trade with India: it suspended trade when India revoked Kashmir's semi-autonomous status in 2019. The decision to resume trade did not go far and the Pakistani government reinstated the suspension, suggesting that the prospect of regional cooperation involving both India and Pakistan remains low.

One of the pandemic's severest impact was on travel and tourism: as a tourism and export-dependent economy, Sri Lanka faced a sharp downturn. Besides tourism, Sri Lanka's economy depends on textile, mining and tea and other plantations. Remittances also contribute substantially to the economy. Exports and imports of goods and services made up 23.1% and 29.3% of Sri Lanka's GDP in 2017.[28] Its economy had already been slowing down when Covid-19 arrived. From 5% in 2015, its GDP growth had fallen to 2.3% in 2019, eventually contracting by 3.6% in 2020. The impact on tourism was stark: in 2019, tourism, as a sector, made up 10.4% of Sri Lanka's GDP; in 2020, that figure contracted by 55.6% and stood at 4.9%.[29] In addition, between 2019 and 2020 24.1% jobs in the sector were lost as a result of the pandemic-related travel restrictions. A second source of impact emerged from the slowdown in ready-made garment sector, which employs directly and indirectly between 300,000 and 600,000 workers.[30] Like everywhere else in South Asia, the poverty rate was estimated to have increased: from 9.2% in 2019 to 11.7% in 2020. Although worker migration from Sri

Lanka fell by 56 % during the first half of 2020 compared to 2019, remittances recovered after an initial decline in March and April, continuing the trend during the rest of the year.[31] Sri Lanka, however, faces long-term vulnerability as it has high debt financing challenges and will be vulnerable to external shocks. The World Bank expects a modest recovery in 2021; however, the risks to long-term recovery depend on the global conditions such as garment markets, particularly in the European Union, vaccine administration both in the country and in the economies that send tourists to it and other factors.

Cooperation in South Asia

As the widespread economic distress in the region reached crisis levels in some countries, India used both bilateral and regional means to assist its neighbors. From the standpoint of regional cooperation, the headlining event was the virtual meeting of SAARC leaders on March 15, 2020. Prime Minister Modi proposed and convened the meeting to develop a strategy to combat the pandemic.[32] All SAARC heads of state or government except Pakistan's joined the Indian Prime Minister; Pakistan was represented by its State Minister of Health, Zafar Mirza. At the meeting, Modi suggested establishing a Covid-19 Emergency Fund for and by SAARC members and committed $10 million to it, suggesting that others should contribute voluntarily.[33] Subsequently, all the other countries committed amounts ranging between $100,000 (Bhutan) and $5 million (Sri Lanka). Pakistan pledged $3 million on the condition that the funds be administered by the SAARC Secretariat in Kathmandu.[34] Under the terms of the Fund, a country seeking assistance from it had to submit their requests through the Indian embassy. Given the voluntary nature of the contributions, the SAARC Secretariat opted to keep itself out of the fund's administration. India convened a second meeting of SAARC senior trade officials in April 2020 to gauge the impact of the pandemic on regional trade.[35] Again, all countries except Pakistan sent their representatives. At the March meeting, Pakistan raised India's August 2019 revocation of Article 370 of the Indian constitution, an article that granted special status to the state of Jammu and Kashmir.[36] Pakistan has continued to link this issue to normalizing trade with India in cotton and sugar, now under suspension for over two years. Covid-19 related assistance channeled through the Covid-19 Emergency Fund was, therefore, the only SAARC framework-based effort during the pandemic besides the two currency swaps negotiated between India and Maldives and between India and Sri Lanka.

The SAARC Currency Swap Framework was operationalized in November 2012 to address short term liquidity issues and balance of payments problems until more longer-term arrangements could be made.[37] Maldives and Sri Lanka, both tourism-dependent regional economies, faced harsh economic slow-downs as soon as the pandemic hit. At the time, the Reserve Bank of India, India's central bank, signed a currency swap agreement with Sri Lanka's central bank in the amount of $400 million. Under the agreement, the Central Bank of Sri Lanka could draw US dollars, euros and Indian rupees in multiple tranches up to a limit of $400 million, with the arrangement remaining in effect until November 2020. In May 2020 Sri Lanka requested India for an additional currency swap arrangement of up to $1.1 billion.[38] When the outbreak of the pandemic and the subsequent lockdowns limited travel, leading to a drying up of foreign exchange inflow into Maldives, another tourism-dependent economy, the island state took advantage of a currency swap arrangement signed in July 2019 to access $150 million in April 2020.[39] This swap arrangement was renewed and then repaid early in 2021. Subsequently, Maldives availed of a $250 million swap arrangement with India in January 2021.[40]

Cooperation in Vaccine Procurement and Health

Much of the cooperation that has taken place in the aftermath of the outbreak of the pandemic has been within bilateral frameworks with each of the countries in the region. Immediately after the pandemic erupted and countries in the region went into lockdown, India sent 5.5 tons of essential medicines and a fourteen member Covid-19 Rapid Response Team of medical personnel to Maldives to help with the pandemic. Subsequently, on Maldives' request, India sent another 6.2 tons of essential medicines and hospital consumables such as catheters and nebulizers.[41]

Bangladesh received Covid-19 vaccines from India as a gift and also purchased vaccines from India. In January 2021 Bangladesh received its first supply of 20 million doses of the Oxford/Astra Zeneca Covishield vaccine; this came as a gift from India's neighborhood plus policy. When Prime Minister Narendra Modi visited Bangladesh in March 2021 to celebrate the fiftieth year of Bangladesh's independence, he brought with him another 12 million doses as a gift. In addition, Bangladesh purchased 30 million doses of this vaccine under a memorandum of understanding that the Bangladesh government and Beximco Pharmaceuticals signed with the Serum Institute, the Indian vaccine manufacturer in December 2020.

Nepal also received 1 million doses of vaccine from India as a gift in January and March of 2021. It made arrangements that had it relying on a commercial agreement for supply of 2 million doses of vaccines from the Serum Institute of India. It also sought to secure some additional doses from the WHO-supported COVAX facility.[42] However, as the second deadly wave of the pandemic unfolded in April–May 2021 and the government faced criticism from the opposition and others, India placed a moratorium on the export of vaccines. When India resumed vaccine exports after a six-month hiatus, Bangladesh and Nepal were among the four countries to which the first shipments were sent.[43]

The surge in Covid-19 cases in India in April 2021 created uncertainty over the availability of vaccines to neighboring countries. When the positive cases increased dramatically, leaders of India's opposition parties demanded an immediate halt on all vaccine exports, so that Indian citizens had access to vaccines first. This led all of India's neighbors to look for other sources of supply and created an opportunity for China. While India's early actions in 2020 earned it plaudits, the unfolding crisis surrounding the second wave did substantial damage to India's reputation.

An Opportunity for China

The outbreak of the Covid-19 pandemic in Wuhan, China, the mystery surrounding its origins and China's lack of transparency and cooperation in uncovering it led many countries, including those in South Asia, to be distrustful of China during the early months following the pandemic's outbreak. Furthermore, Sinovac's relatively limited efficacy meant that countries were not eager to source their vaccines from China. In comparison, India's reputation as the vaccine factory of the world, the Serum Institute of India's collaboration with AstraZeneca and researchers from Oxford University, combined with the vaccine's higher efficacy and lower price made it the vaccine of choice among developing countries. As mentioned in the previous section, India's sudden halting of vaccine exports opened up an opportunity for China. While China had not been entirely absent from South Asia after the pandemic spread, now it was able to leverage its vaccine and its deep pockets to further entrench its position in the region. Here, the chapter shows how China was able to take advantage of India's faltering vaccine policy to increase its profile in the region.

Sri Lanka's dependence on China has significantly increased since the outbreak of the pandemic. Sri Lanka was already facing a large debt burden when Covid-19 brought its economy to a crisis. In March 2020 China announced a $500 million loan to Sri Lanka to help the latter battle the effect of the virus. According to IMF estimates, as a result of a tanking tourism sector and other factors, Sri Lanka's net borrowings were likely to rise to 9.4% of its GDP in 2020, up from 6.8% in 2019.[44] The government asked its employees to give up a part or the entire amount of their salaries to cover the gap in the budget. China was already a big creditor: an estimated 9–15% of Sri Lanka's debt was owed to China. In April 2021 Sri Lanka entered another agreement with the China Development Bank for another $500 million loan. In between these two, there were other loans and a $1.5 billion currency swap deal.[45] This was part of the deal signed in the previous year and was necessitated by a precarious drop in Sri Lanka's foreign exchange reserves to $4.05 billion, a low not seen since the global financial crisis a decade earlier. At the same time, Sri Lanka has an annual debt repayment obligation to the tune of $4.5 billion until 2025.[46]

China reached out to Bangladesh, Nepal and others as well. In May 2020 the Chinese-led Asian Infrastructure Investment Bank approved a $250 million loan to Bangladesh to help the latter to fight the pandemic.[47] The loan, co-financed by the Asian Development Bank, was aimed at strengthening social safety nets and addressing the impact of job losses in small and medium enterprises and in the informal sector, where the most vulnerable are employed. In April 2021 China hosted a meeting of South Asian foreign ministers as the Covid-19 second wave peaked in India. Among other efforts to cooperate on fighting the pandemic, China suggested setting up coronavirus vaccine storage facilities in the region. As the demand in India to restrict vaccine exports grew, China offered to sell Covid-19 vaccines to Bangladesh. Around the same time, it also promised 1million doses of vaccines as a grant assistance to Nepal, which was facing a shortage of vaccines amid a deadly second wave.[48] After 800,000 doses were delivered, the government of Nepal sought to procure 4 million more doses for an undisclosed price.[49] The price of each India-manufactured Covishield dose is $4 while Nepalese media speculated that the price of two Sinovac doses was between $18 and $21.[50] Following the meeting mentioned above, China launched the China-South Asia Emergency Supplies Reserve and Poverty Alleviation and Cooperative Development Centre involving Afghanistan, Bangladesh, Nepal, Pakistan, and Sri Lanka.[51] Bhutan and Maldives did not join.

India has long been the dominant development partner for Bangladesh, Bhutan, Nepal, and Sri Lanka, extending grants and low-interest loans for various projects. In recent years, under the Belt and Road Initiative, China has offered financing and other assistance for infrastructure projects in the region. Several countries in the region have now become wary of China's assistance and intervention. Besides posing a challenge to Indian dominance in the region, these overtures from China have led to outcomes that the citizens of these South Asian countries have come to treat with much suspicion and misgiving. The 2.1-km (1.3 mile) bridge between Malé and its international airport illustrates the sources of such wariness. While the bridge certainly eased transportation issues between the two islands, along with other projects, it left Maldives in as much as $3.1 billion debt to China which helped finance and build the project. This project was initiated under the former pro-Chinese president Abdullah Yameen who was defeated in the 2018 elections. The new government has discovered the extent of indebtedness on account of government-to-government loans, money given to state enterprises and private sector loans guaranteed by the government of Maldives.[52] Former and current officials as well as the Chinese government disagree about the exact sum but given Maldives' $4.9 billion annual GDP, paying back the loan would have been a challenge for Maldives even without the precipitous fall in tourist traffic and consequently, its GDP, on account of the pandemic. Sri Lanka's experience with developing the Hambantota port tells a more alarming story. The Sri Lankan government borrowed from China to develop a port in the coastal town of Hambantota. When Sri Lanka was unable to repay the loans it had taken for the port development, China negotiated a 99-year lease on the port and on 15,000 acres of land around it and effectively gained a foothold in South Asia, a few hundred miles off the Indian coast and along a critical maritime route.[53]

Conclusion

This chapter highlights the challenges and opportunities associated with regional cooperation in South Asia in general and how these have manifested themselves in the context of the Covid-19 pandemic in particular. While in the earlier era, Pakistan's actions and its rivalry with India played a larger role in slowing down cooperation, China's entry into the region's politics and its closer relations with Pakistan now poses a much larger challenge than Pakistan alone posed in the past. This has also initiated a regional competition for power between China and India. Relatedly, past experience and the lack of progress within SAARC in cooperation on trade and other economic issues has moved the discussion on regional cooperation to other sub-regional groups such as BIMSTEC and BBIN, where the focus has been on building connectivity and infrastructure projects rather than on trade liberalization. Against that backdrop, Modi's initiative in setting up the virtual meeting to cooperate on addressing the pandemic was a significant effort to revive region-wide cooperation, given that the outbreak of the pandemic was an excellent example of a crisis around which countries needed to cooperate. However, not only did Pakistan's actions stymie the effort at building a sustainable cooperative effort, India's own inept handling of the second wave provided an opening for China to build an alternative platform. The episode demonstrates, yet again, the need for India to focus on creating a robust framework and capacity for providing regional public goods such as medicines and vaccines along with investments and infrastructure funding. The episode also shows that the government's response to migrant workers's plight during the first wave and the absence of supplies during the second wave tied the government's hand in foreign policy. The halt in exports tarnished India's image as a reliable partner in solving the region's problems. Equally importantly, it left an unmet need that provided China another opportunity. For South Asia, regional cooperation should seek to alleviate poverty and foster economic development. Developmental institutions such as the World Bank suggest that the region should focus on building physical and virtual connectivity and strengthen the quality of human resources instead of waiting for market integration efforts. Creating more robust regional capacity will minimize the necessity for states to look outside for help and to rely on bilateral sources of aid. In August 2021 India invited the SAARC Secretary General to New Delhi for a week to explore avenues to deepen regional cooperation and address the negative impact of the coronavirus pandemic: whether this reflects further thinking on regional cooperation on New Delhi's part remains to be seen.[54]

Notes

1 Instead of defining poverty in monetary terms as used to be the norm, the concept of multidimensional poverty takes into account access to health and education along with standard of living. United Nations Development Program and Oxford Poverty and Human Development Initiative, *Charting pathways out of multidimensional poverty: Achieving the SDGs*, 2020.

2 Constantino Xavier, *Sambandh as Strategy: India's New Approach to Regional Connectivity* (New Delhi, India: Brookings Institution India, 2020).

3 Ibid.

4 For a detailed discussion, see Lok Raj Baral, 'SAARC but no "SHARK": South Asian Regional Cooperation in Perspective', *Pacific Affairs*, 58, no. 3 (Autumn 1985): 411–426.

5 Shivshankar Menon, *India and Asian Geopolitics: The Past, Present* (Washington, DC: Brookings Institution Press, 2021): 179.

6 Pramod Kumar Mishra, 'Dhaka to New Delhi: One Decade of SAARC,' *India Quarterly*, 52, no. ½ (January–June 1996): 74.

7 The Gujral doctrine is a set of five principles of foreign policy that the Indian Prime Minister, Inder Kumar Gujral, articulated during his brief tenure in 1997–98. One of these principles stated that India should not look for reciprocity when dealing with its neighbors. Bhabani Sengupta, 'Security Dimensions of the Gujral Doctrine', Institute of Peace and Conflict Studies, 2 August 1997. www.ipcs.org/focusthemsel.php?articleNo=2.

8 Saman Kalegama, 'Towards Greater Economic Connectivity in South Asia', *Economic and Political Weekly*, 42, no. 39: 3911–3915.

9 Sanjay Kathuria (ed.), *A Glass Half Full: The Promise of Regional Trade in South Asia* (Washington, DC: World Bank, 2019): 35.

10 Dushni Weerakoon and Jayanthi Thennakoon, 'SAFTA: Myth of Free Trade', *Economic and Political Weekly*, 41 (September 16–22, 2006): 3920–3923.

11 Ibid.

12 Kunal Mukherjee, 'The South Asian Association for Regional Cooperation: Problems and Prospects', *Progress in Development Studies*, 14:4 (2014): 373–81; Yogendra Kumar, Amita Batra, Kanwal Sibal and others, 'Debate: Regional Cooperation in South Asia: The Present and The Future', *Indian Foreign Affairs Journal*, 9:4 (2014): 307–50.

13 Jayanth Jacob and Anil Giri, 'SAARC summit collapses after India and three other members pull out', *Hindustan Times*, September 29, 2016. www.hindustantimes.com/world-news/saarc-summit-collapses-after-india-and-3-other-members-pull-out/story-kIMWfSqirGLzB6MEfuS3CN.html.

14 Christoph Lakner et al, 'Updated estimates of the impact of COVID-19 on global poverty: Looking back at 2020 and the outlook for 2021', World Bank, https://blogs.worldbank.org/opendata/updated-estimates-impact-COVID-19-global-poverty-looking-back-2020-and-outlook-2021#:~:text=Using%20the%20growth%20forecast%20from,each%20contributing%20roughly%20two%2Dfifths.

15 International Monetary Fund. 2020. "Helping Bangladesh Recover from COVID-19." *IMF Country Focus*, June, www.imf.org/en/News/Articles/2020/06/11/na-06122020-helping-bangladesh-recover-from-COVID-19.

16 'Bangladesh: Overview', World Bank, www.worldbank.org/en/country/bangladesh/overview#1.

17 World Bank, 'Bangladesh Development Update – Moving Forward: Connectivity and Logistics to strengthen Competitiveness' https://pubdocs.worldbank.org/en/208851617818495059/Bangladesh-Development-Update-Spring-2021.pdf.

18 'Wage Earners Remittance Inflows: Selected Country wise (Monthly)', Bangladesh Bank www.bb.org.bd/econdata/wagermidtl.php.

19 Author's calculation based on data from the World Bank and the Bangladesh Bank, the country's central bank.

20 Bangladesh Bank, 'Monthly data of Wage earner's remittance', www.bb.org.bd/econdata/wageremitance.php.

21 Bangladesh Bank, 'Yearly data of Wage earner's remittance', www.bb.org.bd/econdata/wageremitance.php#.

22 *World Bank, Beaten or Broken: Informality and COVID-19*, South Asia Economic Focus, Fall 2020, 117.

23 Ibid.

24 Sangam Prasain, 'Tourism is Nepal's fourth largest industry by employment, analytical study shows', *The Kathmandu Post*, June 17, 2021. https://kathmandup ost.com/money/2021/06/17/tourism-is-nepal-s-fourth-largest-industry-by-employm ent-study.

25 World Bank, *South Asia Vaccinates*, South Asia Economic Focus, Spring 2021, 193.

26 'Impact Assessment of COVID-19 on Pakistan's Manufacturing Firms, UNIDO, March 2021. www.unido.org/sites/default/files/files/2021-03/UNIDO%20COVID19 %20Assessment_Pakistan_FINAL.pdf.

27 World Bank, *South Asia Vaccinates*, p. 195.

28 'Sri Lanka trade statistics', World Integrated Trade Solution, World Bank, 2021. https://wits.worldbank.org/CountryProfile/en/LKA.

29 World Travel and Tourism Council, 'Sri Lanka, 2020 Annual Research: Key Highlights' https://wttc.org/Research/Economic-Impact.

30 'Securing Women's Place in Sri Lanka's Apparel Industry', Development Asia, Asian Development Bank, August 31, 2020 https://development.asia/insight/secur ing-womens-place-sri-lankas-apparel-industry.

31 Bilesha Weeraratne, 'How Sri Lankan remittances are defying COVID-19,'East Asia Forum, January 28, 2021. www.eastasiaforum.org/2021/01/28/how-sri-lanka n-remittances-are-defying-COVID-19.

32 Elizabeth Roche, 'Coronavirus: Modi calls for SAARC nations' conference to build strategy', *Mint*, March 13, 2020.

33 'PM Modi proposes COVID-19 emergency fund to SAARC leaders, offers $10 mn', *Mint*, March 15, 2020.

34 Arindam Roy, 'Saarc COVID fund: No Indian money for Pakistan; Nepal biggest beneficiary', *Business Standard*, November 30, 2020.

35 'COVID-19: Pakistan skips second SAARC meeting held to discuss impact on regional trade', Scroll.in, April 8 2020. https://scroll.in/latest/958657/COVID-19- pakistan-skips-second-saarc-meeting-held-to-discuss-impact-on-regional-trade.

36 'PM Modi proposes COVID-19 emergency fund'.

37 Reserve Bank of India, 'RBI Signs Currency Swap Agreement with Central Bank of Sri Lanka', July 27, 2020. www.rbi.org.in/scripts/BS_PressReleaseDisplay.aspx? prid=50129.

38 Elizabeth Roche, 'Sri Lanka requests India for currency swap arrangement of up to $1.1 billion', *Mint*, May 23, 2020.

39 Ministry of External Affairs, 'India-Maldives Bilateral Relations', September 2020. https://mea.gov.in/Portal/ForeignRelation/Maldive2020.pdf.

40 Reserve Bank of India, 'Report on Management of Foreign Exchange Reserves', May 12, 2021. www.rbi.org.in/Scripts/PublicationsView.aspx?id=20359.

41 *Financial Express*, 'Operation Sanjeevani: IAF airlifts medical and hospital consum- ables for the Maldives', April 2, 2020. www.financialexpress.com/defence/operation-sa njeevani-iaf-airlifts-medical-and-hospital-consumables-for-the-maldives/1917317.

42 *Hindustan Times*, 'China will donate 1 million doses of COVID-19 vaccines to Nepal: President Xi Jinping', May 26, 2021. www.hindustantimes.com/world-news/china-will- donate-1-million-doses-of-COVID-19-vaccines-to-nepal-president-xi-jinping-101622042 234269.html.

43 *Times of India*, 'India exports COVID-19 vaccine doses to Myanmar, Nepal, Ban- gladesh Iran', October 10, 2021. https://timesofindia.indiatimes.com/india/india -exports-COVID-19-vaccine-doses-to-myanmar-nepal-bangladesh-iran/articleshow/ 86909125.cms.

44 Munza Mushtaq, 'Sri Lanka piles on more Chinese loans amid virus and debt crisis', May 15, 2020.

https://asia.nikkei.com/Politics/International-relations/Sri-Lanka-piles-on-more-Chinese-loans-amid-virus-and-debt-crisis.

45 *Times of India*, 'China Development Bank extends 500 million loan to Sri Lanka', April 12, 2021. https://timesofindia.indiatimes.com/world/china/china-developm ent-bank-to-extend-500-million-loan-to-sri-lanka/articleshow/82034712.cms.

46 *Business Standard*, 'Sri Lanka signs three year 1.5 billion currency swap deal with China', March 23 2021. www.business-standard.com/article/international/sri-lanka-signs-three-year-1-5-billion-currency-swap-deal-with-china-121032300053_1.html.

47 Reuters, 'China-backed AIIB approves $250 million loan for Bangladesh's COVID-19 response', May 20, 2020. www.reuters.com/article/us-health-corona virus-aiib-bangladesh/china-backed-aiib-approves-250-million-loan-for-bangladeshs-COVID-19-response-idUSKBN22X08Z.

48 *Hindustan Times*, 'China will donate 1 million doses of COVID-19 vaccines to Nepal: President Xi Jinping', May 26, 2021. www.hindustantimes.com/world-news/china-will-donate-1-million-doses-of-COVID-19-vaccines-to-nepal-president-xi-jinping-1016 22042234269.html.

49 *Business Standard*, 'Nepal to procure 4 million COVID vaccines from China under non-disclosure deal', June 17, 2021. www.business-standard.com/article/current-affairs/nepa l-to-procure-4-mn-COVID-vaccines-from-china-under-non-disclosure-deal-1210617005 60_1.html.

50 Mint, 'China unhappy with Nepal over disclosure of COVID vaccine price', June 20, 2021. https://www.livemint.com/news/world/china-unhappy-with-nepal-over-disclosure-of-sinopharm-covid-vaccine-price-11624146501724.html.

51 Bipin Ghimire and Apoorva Pathak, 'China is Providing an Alternative Regional Framework for South Asia,' *The Diplomat*, July 30, 2021, https://thediplomat.com/2021/07/china-is-providing-an-alternative-regional-framework-for-south-asia.

52 Anbarasan Ethirajan, 'China debt dogs Maldives' 'bridge to prosperity'', September 2020. www.bbc.com/news/world-asia-52743072.

53 Maria Abi-Habib, 'How China Got Sri Lanka to Cough Up a Port', *The New York Times*, June 25, 2018, www.nytimes.com/2018/06/25/world/asia/china-sri-lanka -port.html.

54 'SAARC secretary-general Weerakoon on week-long visit to India to deepen regional cooperation', The Print.in, 8 August 2021. https://theprint.in/diplomacy/saarc-secretary-general-weerakoon-on-week-long-visit-to-india-to-deepen-regional-cooperation/711463.

Index

Page numbers in italics indicate a figure and page numbers in bold indicate a table on the corresponding page.

For Product Safety Concerns and Information please contact our EU
representative GPSR@taylorandfrancis.com
Taylor & Francis Verlag GmbH, Kaufingerstraße 24, 80331 München, Germany